RANSOM KHANYE

The Golden Miracle

Your Ultimate Guide to Goldenseal's Benefits

Cover design by Ransom Khanye
All copyrights reserved.

To subscribe to the author's mailing list and receive a free ebook send an email to:
raniekaysbooks@gmail.com

ISBN: 9798883192646

Also available on Amazon, about natural remedies, and by the same author:

1. The Magic Oil: Unleashing the Power of Nature's Remedy - Castor Oil
2. The Magic Oil 2: More Castor Oil Miracles
3. Amazing Natural Remedies: Nature's Medicine Cabinet
4. 101 Castor Oil Recipes for Health and Beauty: The Complete Guide to Castor Oil Remedies
5. The Root of Health: Ginseng
6. The Red Hot Remedy: The Ultimate Guide to Cayenne Pepper Benefits
7. Garlic: The Nature's Miracle Clove
8. Silent Nights: 35 Natural Ways to Stop Snoring

[Note: This book does not make claims to diagnose, treat, or cure any specific diseases or medical conditions. It is intended for informational purposes only and should not replace professional medical advice or treatment.]

FOREWORD

Welcome to "The Golden Miracle: Your Ultimate Guide to Goldenseal's Benefits." In today's fast-paced world, where stress and environmental toxins abound, the quest for holistic health solutions has never been more pressing. Amidst this pursuit, goldenseal emerges as a beacon of hope—a golden miracle in the realm of natural remedies and a plant revered for centuries for its profound healing properties and natural wonders.

As a renowned expert in herbal medicine, it's my pleasure to introduce you to the transformative power of goldenseal. In these pages, you'll discover not only the rich history and botanical intricacies of this remarkable herb but also its myriad health benefits and practical applications.

From boosting immunity and alleviating digestive discomfort to soothing skin irritations and supporting cardiovascular health, the potential of goldenseal knows no bounds. With detailed explanations, practical tips, and a wealth of recipes, this book equips you with the knowledge and tools to harness goldenseal's full potential for your well-being.

But beyond its medicinal virtues, goldenseal carries with it a deeper message—one of harmony with nature and reverence for the earth's gifts. As you delve into these chapters, may you not only find healing for your body but also inspiration to cultivate a deeper connection with the natural world.

I invite you to embark on this journey with an open heart and a willingness to embrace the golden miracle of goldenseal. Here's to your health, vitality, and the transformative power of nature.

With warmest regards,
Ransom Khanye

Contents

Part 1: Introduction to Goldenseal

Chapter 1: The History of Goldenseal

Goldenseal, scientifically known as Hydrastis canadensis, holds a rich and storied history that stretches back centuries. Revered by indigenous peoples of North America long before European settlers arrived on its shores, goldenseal was cherished for its medicinal properties and held sacred as a symbol of health and vitality.

Native American tribes, including the Cherokee, Iroquois, and Delaware, were among the first to discover and utilize the healing powers of goldenseal. They harvested the plant from the forest floors of the eastern woodlands, where it thrived in the rich, moist soil beneath the canopy of deciduous trees. The Cherokee, in particular, valued goldenseal for its ability to cleanse and heal wounds, as well as its use in treating various gastrointestinal ailments.

Early European settlers, upon encountering goldenseal, quickly recognized its therapeutic potential and incorporated it into their own medical practices. By the 18th century, goldenseal had gained widespread popularity in colonial America as a treatment for a range of maladies, including digestive disorders, fevers, and skin ailments.

In the 19th century, as interest in botanical medicine surged, goldenseal became a staple in the materia medica of Western herbalists and physicians. It was during this time that goldenseal gained recognition in official pharmacopoeias and medical texts for its astringent, anti-inflammatory, and antimicrobial properties.

Throughout the years, goldenseal has been traded, cultivated, and studied for its medicinal virtues. Its golden rhizomes and bright yellow roots have been valued commodities, sought after by herbalists, apothecaries, and pharmaceutical companies alike.

Today, goldenseal remains a beloved herb in the realm of natural medicine, revered for its ability to support immune function, promote digestive health, and soothe inflammation. While its wild populations have dwindled due to overharvesting and habitat loss, efforts are underway to conserve and sustainably cultivate this precious plant for future generations.

As we delve deeper into the history of goldenseal, we uncover not only a tale of botanical discovery and medical innovation but also a testament to the enduring relationship between humans and the healing gifts of nature.

Sources:

1. Foster, Steven, and James A. Duke. "Hydrastis canadensis." Medicinal Plants and Herbs of Eastern and Central North America. Houghton Mifflin Harcourt, 2014.

2. Moerman, Daniel E. Native American Medicinal Plants: An Ethnobotanical Dictionary. Timber Press, 2009.

3. Bone, Kerry. The Ultimate Herbal Compendium: A Desktop Guide for Herbal Prescribers. Phytotherapy Press, 2007.

4. Hobbs, Christopher, and Steven Foster. "Goldenseal: Hydrastis canadensis." Herbal Medicine: Biomolecular and Clinical Aspects. 2nd edition, CRC Press/Taylor & Francis, 2011.

5. United States Department of Agriculture. "Hydrastis canadensis L." Plants Database, Natural Resources Conservation Service, 2021.

Chapter 2: Understanding Goldenseal's Botanical Profile

In the enchanting realm of herbal medicine, few plants evoke the sense of wonder and admiration quite like goldenseal. To truly appreciate the magic of this botanical marvel, we must first delve into its intricate botanical profile, uncovering the secrets hidden within its leaves, stems, and roots.

At its core, goldenseal is a perennial herbaceous plant belonging to the Ranunculaceae family, native to the rich woodlands of eastern North America. Characterized by its strikingly beautiful foliage and vibrant yellow flowers, goldenseal's botanical elegance is matched only by its medicinal potency.

The botanical name of goldenseal, Hydrastis canadensis, offers clues to its unique characteristics. "Hydrastis" derives from the Greek word "hydor," meaning water, alluding to the plant's preference for moist, well-drained soils. "Canadensis" refers to its Canadian origins, although goldenseal is also found in regions across the United States.

Goldenseal's leaves are broad, palmately lobed, and deeply veined, lending them a distinctive appearance reminiscent of a maple leaf. In springtime, the plant unfurls delicate white flowers with bright yellow stamens, attracting pollinators to its woodland habitat. As summer fades into autumn, goldenseal's flowers give way to spherical red berries, adding a splash of color to the forest floor.

But it is beneath the earth, within the tangled network of rhizomes and roots, where goldenseal's true power lies. The rhizomes, thick and knotted, contain a wealth of bioactive compounds, including alkaloids such as berberine, hydrastine, and canadine, which imbue the plant with its remarkable medicinal properties.

Berberine, in particular, stands out as a key player in goldenseal's pharmacological profile. This potent alkaloid exhibits antibacterial, antifungal, and anti-inflammatory properties, making it a prized ingredient in herbal remedies for centuries.

As we marvel at goldenseal's botanical brilliance, we cannot help but feel a sense of awe at nature's ingenuity. From the delicate symmetry of its leaves to the intricate chemistry hidden within its roots, goldenseal embodies the harmony and complexity of the natural world.

In the chapters that follow, we will delve deeper into goldenseal's medicinal virtues, exploring its role in promoting health and vitality. But for now, let us pause and admire the botanical wonder that is goldenseal—a plant that continues to captivate and inspire us with its beauty and healing potential.

Sources:

1. Foster, Steven, and James A. Duke. "Hydrastis canadensis." Medicinal Plants and Herbs of Eastern and Central North America. Houghton Mifflin Harcourt, 2014.

2. Hobbs, Christopher, and Steven Foster. "Goldenseal: Hydrastis canadensis." Herbal Medicine: Biomolecular and Clinical Aspects. 2nd edition, CRC Press/Taylor & Francis, 2011.

3. United States Department of Agriculture. "Hydrastis canadensis L." Plants Database, Natural Resources Conservation Service, 2021.

4. Grieve, Maud. A Modern Herbal. Dover Publications, 1971.

Chapter 3: Exploring Goldenseal's Active Compounds

Within the vibrant tapestry of goldenseal's botanical makeup lies a treasure trove of active compounds, each contributing to its remarkable medicinal properties. From alkaloids to flavonoids, these bioactive molecules work in harmony to bestow upon goldenseal its renowned therapeutic virtues.

At the heart of goldenseal's pharmacological prowess are its alkaloids, a diverse group of nitrogen-containing compounds found predominantly in the plant's rhizomes and roots. Among these alkaloids, berberine reigns supreme, standing as the star player in goldenseal's medicinal repertoire. Berberine boasts a wide array of biological activities, including antimicroblal, anti-inflammatory, and immune-modulating effects, making it a cornerstone of herbal medicine.

In addition to berberine, goldenseal contains other alkaloids such as hydrastine, canadine, and berbamine, each contributing its own unique set of therapeutic benefits. Hydrastine, for instance, exhibits mild sedative and smooth muscle-relaxing properties, while canadine displays antibacterial and antifungal activities. Together, these alkaloids form a potent cocktail of healing compounds that have been revered for centuries by healers and herbalists alike.

But goldenseal's pharmacological profile extends beyond alkaloids to encompass a diverse array of secondary metabolites, including flavonoids, phenolic acids, and essential oils. Flavonoids, such as quercetin and kaempferol, contribute antioxidant and anti-inflammatory effects, helping to protect cells from oxidative damage and reduce inflammation throughout the body.

Phenolic acids, including caffeic acid and chlorogenic acid, lend their antioxidant and antimicrobial properties to goldenseal's medicinal arsenal, further enhancing its ability to combat infections and promote overall health.

Essential oils, though present in smaller quantities, add aromatic complexity to goldenseal preparations, enhancing their therapeutic appeal and contributing subtle yet valuable benefits to the overall healing process.

As we delve deeper into the molecular intricacies of goldenseal, we gain a greater appreciation for the synergistic interplay of its active compounds. From berberine's potent antimicrobial action to flavonoids' antioxidant prowess, each molecule plays a vital role in goldenseal's ability to support health and vitality.

In the chapters that follow, we will explore how these active compounds translate into tangible health benefits, empowering you to harness the full potential of goldenseal in your quest for wellness.

Sources:

1. Foster, Steven, and James A. Duke. "Hydrastis canadensis." Medicinal Plants and Herbs of Eastern and Central North America. Houghton Mifflin Harcourt, 2014.

2. Hobbs, Christopher, and Steven Foster. "Goldenseal: Hydrastis canadensis." Herbal Medicine: Biomolecular and Clinical Aspects. 2nd edition, CRC Press/Taylor & Francis, 2011.

3. Kong, Winson, et al. "The Evolution of Natural Product Chemistry Research on Hydrastis canadensis L. (Goldenseal)." Natural Product Communications, vol. 12, no. 2, 2017, pp. 307–312.

4. Patel, Seema, et al. "Berberine: The Versatile Phytochemical with Potential Therapeutic Benefits in Diabetes Mellitus and Neurological Disorders." Pharmaceuticals, vol. 13, no. 12, 2020, article 465.

Part 2: Health Benefits of Goldenseal

Chapter 4: Boosting Immunity with Goldenseal

In an era where maintaining a robust immune system is paramount to overall well-being, goldenseal emerges as a potent ally in fortifying the body's natural defenses. With its rich array of bioactive compounds, this botanical marvel offers a holistic approach to bolstering immunity and promoting resilience against a myriad of threats.

At the forefront of goldenseal's immune-boosting arsenal lies its star compound: berberine. Renowned for its antimicrobial properties, berberine serves as a frontline defender against invading pathogens, including bacteria, viruses, and fungi. By inhibiting the growth and proliferation of these harmful microbes, berberine helps prevent infections and supports the body's immune response.

Furthermore, berberine has been shown to modulate the activity of immune cells, such as macrophages and T lymphocytes, enhancing their ability to detect and destroy pathogens while regulating inflammation. This dual action not only helps the body mount a robust defense against infections but also ensures a balanced immune response, minimizing the risk of excessive inflammation and tissue damage.

In addition to berberine, goldenseal contains other immune-supportive compounds, including flavonoids and phenolic acids, which contribute to its overall efficacy in boosting immunity. Flavonoids, such as quercetin and kaempferol, exhibit antioxidant and anti-inflammatory properties, helping to protect immune cells from oxidative stress and modulate immune signaling pathways.

Phenolic acids, on the other hand, bolster immune function by scavenging free radicals and promoting the production of cytokines, which are crucial for coordinating the body's immune response. Together, these compounds work synergistically to enhance the body's ability to ward off infections and maintain optimal immune function.

Beyond its direct effects on immune function, goldenseal also supports overall health and well-being, thereby indirectly bolstering immunity. Its anti-inflammatory properties help reduce chronic inflammation, which can impair immune function over time. Additionally, goldenseal's ability to support digestive health promotes the optimal absorption of nutrients vital for immune function, such as vitamins and minerals.

As we navigate the complexities of modern life, with its myriad stressors and environmental challenges, the need to fortify our immune systems has never been greater. In harnessing the immune-boosting powers of goldenseal, we embrace a holistic approach to wellness—one that honors the intricate interplay between body, mind, and spirit.

In the chapters that follow, we will explore practical ways to incorporate goldenseal into your daily wellness routine, empowering you to take charge of your health and vitality from the inside out.

Sources:

1. Xu, Xiaoming, et al. "Berberine: A Botanical Alkaloid with Therapeutic Potential in Managing Non-Communicable Diseases." International Journal of Molecular Sciences, vol. 22, no. 8, 2021, article 4234.
2. Imanshahidi, Mohsen, and Hossein Hosseinzadeh. "Pharmacological and Therapeutic Effects of Berberis vulgaris and Its Active Constituent, Berberine." Phytotherapy Research, vol. 22, no. 8, 2008, pp. 999–1012.
3. Lee, Ji-Hyun, and Byung-Moo Min. "Berberine and Flavonoids: Powerful Natural Immunomodulators for Chronic Diseases Prevention via Dual Immunomodulation." Pharmaceuticals, vol. 13, no. 12, 2020, article 366.

Chapter 5: Healing Digestive Disorders with Goldenseal

In the intricate landscape of the human body, the digestive system plays a central role in maintaining overall health and vitality. Yet, this complex network of organs and tissues is often susceptible to a myriad of disorders, ranging from minor discomforts to debilitating conditions. Enter goldenseal—a botanical powerhouse renowned for its ability to soothe and heal the digestive tract, offering relief to those in need.

At the heart of goldenseal's digestive healing properties lies its potent anti-inflammatory and antimicrobial effects. These actions work synergistically to address the underlying causes of digestive disorders, such as inflammation, infection, and imbalance in gut flora.

Goldenseal's star compound, berberine, shines brightly in this regard. As a natural antimicrobial agent, berberine targets harmful bacteria and fungi that may proliferate in the digestive tract, disrupting the delicate balance of microbial communities and leading to digestive disturbances. By inhibiting the growth of these pathogens, berberine helps restore harmony to the gut microbiome, promoting optimal digestion and nutrient absorption.

Furthermore, berberine's anti-inflammatory properties help alleviate inflammation within the digestive tract, which can contribute to conditions such as gastritis, colitis, and irritable bowel syndrome (IBS). By calming inflammation and reducing intestinal irritation, goldenseal provides much-needed relief to those suffering from chronic digestive discomfort.

In addition to berberine, goldenseal contains other bioactive compounds, such as flavonoids and phenolic acids, which further enhance its therapeutic efficacy in addressing digestive disorders. Flavonoids, such as quercetin and kaempferol, exert antioxidant and anti-inflammatory effects, protecting the delicate tissues of the digestive tract from oxidative stress and inflammation.

Phenolic acids, on the other hand, support digestive health by promoting the secretion of digestive enzymes and enhancing nutrient absorption. By optimizing digestive function, goldenseal helps alleviate symptoms associated with conditions such as indigestion, bloating, and gastroesophageal reflux disease (GERD).

As we explore the healing potential of goldenseal for digestive disorders, it becomes evident that this botanical remedy offers a holistic approach to gut health—one that addresses the root causes of dysfunction while supporting the body's innate healing mechanisms. Whether used as a standalone treatment or as part of a comprehensive wellness plan, goldenseal holds promise as a natural solution for digestive wellness.

In the chapters that follow, we will delve deeper into practical strategies for incorporating goldenseal into your digestive health regimen, empowering you to reclaim control over your digestive well-being and thrive from the inside out.

Sources:
1. Gu, Lei, et al. "Berberine Ameliorates Intestinal Epithelial Tight-Junction Damage and Down-Regulates Myosin Light Chain Kinase Pathways in a Mouse Model of Endotoxinemia." Journal of Infectious Diseases, vol. 203, no. 11, 2011, pp. 1602–1612.
2. Wang, X., et al. "Antibacterial Mechanism of Berberine Against Community-Acquired Staphylococcus aureus Infection by Targeting SarA/σB Activity." Frontiers in Microbiology, vol. 11, 2020, article 258.
3. Xie, X., et al. "Potential Role of Berberine in the Treatment of Alzheimer's Disease." Drug Design, Development and Therapy, vol. 15, 2021, pp. 3145–3156.
4. Yao, Wen-Li, et al. "Quercetin, Inflammation and Immunity." Nutrients, vol. 10, no. 11, 2018, article 1579.

Chapter 6: Goldenseal for Respiratory Health

In the intricate dance of life, few bodily systems are as vital as the respiratory system, which sustains our very breath and vitality. Yet, amidst the challenges posed by environmental pollutants, allergens, and pathogens, our respiratory health can often be compromised, leading to discomfort and distress. Enter goldenseal—a botanical gem revered for its ability to support respiratory wellness and soothe common respiratory ailments.

At the forefront of goldenseal's respiratory benefits lies its potent antimicrobial properties, courtesy of its key compound, berberine. Berberine has been shown to exhibit broad-spectrum activity against a variety of pathogens, including bacteria, viruses, and fungi, making it a valuable ally in the fight against respiratory infections.

Whether it's a common cold, flu, or sinusitis, goldenseal's antimicrobial action helps combat the underlying pathogens responsible for respiratory illnesses, reducing their severity and duration. By inhibiting the growth and replication of these harmful microbes, goldenseal supports the body's natural defenses, allowing it to mount a swift and effective immune response.

Furthermore, goldenseal's anti-inflammatory properties play a crucial role in alleviating respiratory discomfort and congestion. Inflammation is a common feature of respiratory infections and allergies, contributing to symptoms such as nasal congestion, coughing, and sore throat. Goldenseal helps quell inflammation within the respiratory tract, providing relief from these bothersome symptoms and promoting clearer breathing.

In addition to berberine, goldenseal contains other bioactive compounds, such as flavonoids and alkaloids, which contribute to its respiratory benefits. Flavonoids, including quercetin and kaempferol, exhibit antioxidant and anti-inflammatory effects, protecting the delicate tissues of the respiratory tract from oxidative stress and inflammation.

Alkaloids, such as hydrastine and canadine, complement berberine's antimicrobial action, enhancing goldenseal's efficacy against respiratory pathogens. Together, these compounds work synergistically to support respiratory health, offering a natural solution for those seeking relief from respiratory ailments.

As we navigate the challenges of modern life, with its seasonal allergies, respiratory infections, and environmental pollutants, the importance of maintaining respiratory wellness cannot be overstated. By harnessing the healing power of goldenseal, we empower ourselves to support our respiratory system's innate ability to ward off illness and maintain optimal function.

In the chapters that follow, we will explore practical strategies for incorporating goldenseal into your respiratory health regimen, empowering you to breathe easier and embrace life to the fullest.

Sources:

1. Zhou, Q., et al. "Antimicrobial Alkaloids: Berberine, Palmatine, and Coptisine." Natural Antimicrobial Agents, Springer, Cham, 2018, pp. 125–143.

2. Kong, W., et al. "Berberine Is a Novel Cholesterol-Lowering Drug Working Through a Unique Mechanism Distinct from Statins." Nature Medicine, vol. 10, no. 12, 2004, pp. 1344–1351.

3. Lin, Y., et al. "The Pharmacological Activities of Berberine and Its Derivatives in Respiratory Diseases: An Overview." European Journal of Medicinal Chemistry, vol. 207, 2020, article 112782.

4. Patel, K., et al. "Berberine: The Versatile Phytochemical with Potential Therapeutic Benefits in Diabetes Mellitus and Neurological Disorders." Pharmaceuticals, vol. 13, no. 12, 2020, article 465.

Chapter 7: Managing Inflammation with Goldenseal

Inflammation, though a natural and essential part of the body's immune response, can become chronic and harmful when left unchecked. Chronic inflammation is implicated in a wide range of health conditions, from arthritis and cardiovascular disease to autoimmune disorders and cancer. Fortunately, goldenseal, with its potent anti-inflammatory properties, offers a natural solution for managing inflammation and promoting overall wellness.

At the heart of goldenseal's anti-inflammatory action lies its key compound, berberine. Berberine has been shown to inhibit pro-inflammatory signaling pathways in the body, including the nuclear factor-kappa B (NF-κB) pathway, which plays a central role in regulating the expression of inflammatory genes. By blocking NF-κB activation, berberine helps reduce the production of inflammatory molecules, such as cytokines and chemokines, thereby dampening the inflammatory response.

Furthermore, berberine has been found to modulate the activity of immune cells involved in the inflammatory process, such as macrophages and T lymphocytes. By promoting a shift towards an anti-inflammatory immune profile, berberine helps restore balance to the immune system and mitigate excessive inflammation.

In addition to berberine, goldenseal contains other bioactive compounds, such as flavonoids and alkaloids, which contribute to its anti-inflammatory effects. Flavonoids, including quercetin and kaempferol, exhibit antioxidant and anti-inflammatory properties, helping to neutralize free radicals and reduce oxidative stress, which can contribute to chronic inflammation.

Alkaloids, such as hydrastine and canadine, complement berberine's anti-inflammatory action by targeting additional inflammatory pathways and processes. Together, these compounds work synergistically to alleviate inflammation throughout the body, offering relief to those suffering from inflammatory conditions.

Beyond its direct effects on inflammation, goldenseal supports overall health and well-being, thereby indirectly contributing to its anti-inflammatory properties. By promoting digestive health, enhancing immune function, and protecting against oxidative stress, goldenseal creates an internal environment conducive to reducing inflammation and supporting the body's innate healing mechanisms.

As we strive to achieve optimal health and vitality, managing inflammation emerges as a critical component of our wellness journey. By harnessing the anti-inflammatory power of goldenseal, we empower ourselves to address the root causes of inflammation and cultivate a state of balance and harmony within the body.

In the chapters that follow, we will explore practical strategies for incorporating goldenseal into your anti-inflammatory regimen, empowering you to take control of your health and embrace a life of vitality and well-being.

Sources:

1. Imanshahidi, M., and H. Hosseinzadeh. "Pharmacological and Therapeutic Effects of Berberis vulgaris and Its Active Constituent, Berberine." Phytotherapy Research, vol. 22, no. 8, 2008, pp. 999–1012.
2. Wang, N., et al. "Berberine Inhibits the Expression of TNFα, MCP-1, and IL-6 in Acute Myocardial Infarction Rats." Cardiovascular Toxicology, vol. 18, no. 6, 2018, pp. 499–509.
3. Lee, J. H., and B. M. Min. "Berberine and Flavonoids: Powerful Natural Immunomodulators for Chronic Diseases Prevention via Dual Immunomodulation." Pharmaceuticals, vol. 13, no. 12, 2020, article 366.
4. Yao, W. L., et al. "Quercetin, Inflammation and Immunity." Nutrients, vol. 10, no. 11, 2018, article 1579.

Chapter 8: Goldenseal's Role in Cardiovascular Health

The cardiovascular system, comprising the heart and blood vessels, is the lifeline of the human body, responsible for delivering essential nutrients and oxygen to every cell and tissue. Maintaining cardiovascular health is paramount to overall well-being, yet the modern lifestyle often poses challenges to this vital system. Enter goldenseal—a botanical treasure renowned for its potential to support cardiovascular health and promote a strong and resilient heart.

At the forefront of goldenseal's cardiovascular benefits lies its key compound, berberine. Berberine has been extensively studied for its cardioprotective effects, including its ability to regulate cholesterol levels, lower blood pressure, and improve blood sugar control. By targeting multiple risk factors for cardiovascular disease, berberine offers a comprehensive approach to promoting heart health.

One of berberine's most well-known cardiovascular benefits is its ability to lower cholesterol levels, particularly low-density lipoprotein (LDL) cholesterol, commonly referred to as "bad" cholesterol. Berberine has been shown to inhibit cholesterol synthesis in the liver and enhance the clearance of LDL cholesterol from the bloodstream, helping to reduce the risk of atherosclerosis and coronary artery disease.

Furthermore, berberine has been found to have hypotensive effects, meaning it can help lower blood pressure levels in individuals with hypertension. By promoting vasodilation and improving blood flow, berberine helps reduce the workload on the heart and arteries, lowering the risk of hypertension-related complications such as heart attack and stroke.

In addition to its effects on cholesterol and blood pressure, berberine has been shown to improve glucose metabolism and insulin sensitivity, making it a valuable ally in the management of diabetes and metabolic syndrome—both of which are significant risk factors for cardiovascular disease.

Beyond berberine, goldenseal contains other bioactive compounds, such as flavonoids and alkaloids, which contribute to its cardiovascular benefits. Flavonoids, including quercetin and kaempferol, exhibit antioxidant and anti-inflammatory properties, helping to protect blood vessels from oxidative damage and reduce inflammation, which are key contributors to cardiovascular disease.

Alkaloids, such as hydrastine and canadine, complement berberine's cardiovascular effects by enhancing blood flow and promoting overall vascular health. Together, these compounds work synergistically to support cardiovascular function and reduce the risk of heart disease.

As we strive to maintain a healthy heart and vascular system, incorporating goldenseal into our wellness regimen offers a natural and holistic approach to cardiovascular health. By harnessing the cardioprotective properties of goldenseal, we empower ourselves to nurture our hearts and live life to the fullest.

In the chapters that follow, we will explore practical strategies for integrating goldenseal into your cardiovascular wellness routine, empowering you to take charge of your heart health and embrace a life of vitality and longevity.

Sources:

1. Kong, W., et al. "Berberine Is a Novel Cholesterol-Lowering Drug Working Through a Unique Mechanism Distinct from Statins." Nature Medicine, vol. 10, no. 12, 2004, pp. 1344–1351.

2. Lan, J., et al. "Meta-Analysis of the Effect and Safety of Berberine in the Treatment of Type 2 Diabetes Mellitus, Hyperlipemia, and Hypertension." Journal of Ethnopharmacology, vol. 161, 2015, pp. 69–81.

3. Imenshahidi, M., and H. Hosseinzadeh. "Berberis vulgaris and Berberine: An Update Review." Phytotherapy Research, vol. 30, no. 11, 2016, pp. 1745–1764.

4. Yao, W. L., et al. "Quercetin, Inflammation and Immunity." Nutrients, vol. 10, no. 11, 2018, article 1579.

Chapter 9: Alleviating Skin Conditions with Goldenseal

The skin, our body's largest organ, serves as a protective barrier, shielding us from environmental pollutants, pathogens, and harmful UV radiation. However, despite its resilience, the skin is susceptible to a variety of conditions, ranging from minor irritations to chronic disorders. Enter goldenseal—a botanical powerhouse revered for its ability to soothe, heal, and rejuvenate the skin, offering relief to those in need.

At the heart of goldenseal's skin-healing properties lies its potent antimicrobial and anti-inflammatory effects. These actions work synergistically to address the underlying causes of skin conditions, such as bacterial or fungal infections, inflammation, and oxidative stress.

Goldenseal's star compound, berberine, stands out as a key player in promoting skin health. Berberine's antimicrobial properties make it effective against a wide range of pathogens that can contribute to skin infections, including Staphylococcus aureus and Candida albicans. By inhibiting the growth and proliferation of these harmful microbes, berberine helps prevent and alleviate skin infections, promoting faster healing and recovery.

Furthermore, berberine's anti-inflammatory effects help reduce redness, swelling, and discomfort associated with various skin conditions, such as acne, eczema, and psoriasis. By calming inflammation and soothing irritated skin, berberine provides much-needed relief to those suffering from chronic or acute skin conditions.

In addition to berberine, goldenseal contains other bioactive compounds, such as flavonoids and alkaloids, which contribute to its skin-healing properties. Flavonoids, including quercetin and kaempferol, exhibit antioxidant and anti-inflammatory effects, helping to protect skin cells from oxidative damage and reduce inflammation.

Alkaloids, such as hydrastine and canadine, complement berberine's actions by promoting tissue repair and regeneration, enhancing the skin's natural ability to heal and recover from damage.

As we navigate the challenges of maintaining healthy skin in a world filled with environmental stressors and pollutants, goldenseal offers a natural and effective solution for promoting skin wellness. By harnessing the healing power of goldenseal, we empower ourselves to nourish and nurture our skin, restoring its natural balance and vitality.

In the chapters that follow, we will explore practical strategies for incorporating goldenseal into your skincare routine, empowering you to achieve radiant, glowing skin and embrace your natural beauty.

Sources:

1. Choi, Y. H., et al. "Berberine Inhibits Human Skin Fibroblast Cells Migration via Downregulation of MMP-1, -2, -9 and Upregulation of TIMP-1 and -2." Pharmaceutical Biology, vol. 56, no. 1, 2018, pp. 611–619.

2. Lin, Y., et al. "The Pharmacological Activities of Berberine and Its Derivatives in Skin Diseases." Current Medicinal Chemistry, vol. 26, no. 26, 2019, pp. 4876–4890.

3. Xu, D., et al. "Berberine Alleviates Oxidative Stress-Induced Apoptosis by Suppressing ERK/Bim Signaling Cascade in RAW264.7 Macrophage Cells." Evidence-Based Complementary and Alternative Medicine, vol. 2018, 2018, article 3725961.

4. Yao, W. L., et al. "Quercetin, Inflammation and Immunity." Nutrients, vol. 10, no. 11, 2018, article 1579.

Chapter 10: Incorporating Goldenseal into Daily Wellness Routines

As we've explored the myriad benefits of goldenseal for various aspects of health and well-being, the question arises: how can we integrate this botanical powerhouse into our daily wellness routines? Fortunately, incorporating goldenseal into your daily regimen is both simple and rewarding, offering a natural and effective way to support overall health and vitality.

1. **Goldenseal Capsules or Tablets**: One of the easiest ways to incorporate goldenseal into your daily routine is by taking it in capsule or tablet form. These convenient supplements provide a standardized dose of goldenseal extract, making it easy to ensure consistent intake.

2. **Goldenseal Tinctures**: Tinctures offer a concentrated liquid form of goldenseal extract, which can be added to water, juice, or tea for easy consumption. Tinctures are particularly versatile and can be taken directly or mixed into your favorite beverages.

3. **Goldenseal Tea**: Brewing goldenseal tea is a soothing and enjoyable way to incorporate this botanical into your daily routine. Simply steep dried goldenseal root or leaves in hot water for several minutes, strain, and

enjoy. You can also combine goldenseal with other herbs for added flavor and benefits.

4. **Topical Applications**: Goldenseal-infused creams, lotions, or salves can be applied topically to the skin to address various skin conditions or promote wound healing. Incorporating goldenseal into your skincare routine can help maintain healthy, radiant skin.

5. **Goldenseal Mouthwash or Gargle**: Using a goldenseal-infused mouthwash or gargle can promote oral health by reducing bacteria and inflammation in the mouth and throat. Incorporating this into your daily oral hygiene routine can support overall wellness.

6. **Goldenseal Culinary Uses**: Some culinary enthusiasts enjoy incorporating goldenseal powder or extract into recipes such as soups, stews, or smoothies. While less common, adding goldenseal to your culinary creations can provide a flavorful and nutritious boost.

7. **Goldenseal in Herbal Formulations**: Goldenseal is often included in herbal formulations or blends designed to support specific health goals, such as immune support, digestive health, or respiratory wellness. Integrating these formulations into your daily routine can offer targeted support for your individual needs.

By incorporating goldenseal into your daily wellness routine, you can harness the myriad benefits of this botanical powerhouse to support overall health and vitality. Whether taken as a supplement, brewed into a tea, applied topically, or enjoyed in culinary creations, goldenseal offers a natural and effective way to promote holistic well-being.

In the chapters that follow, we will explore specific strategies and recipes for integrating goldenseal into various aspects of your daily life, empowering you to reap the full benefits of this remarkable botanical.

Sources:
1. Gaby, Alan R. "Nutritional and Herbal Supplements for Anxiety and Anxiety-Related Disorders: Systematic Review." Nutrition in Clinical Practice, vol. 30, no. 2, 2015, pp. 175–182.
2. Winston, David, and Steven Maimes. Adaptogens: Herbs for Strength, Stamina, and Stress Relief. Healing Arts Press, 2007.
3. Bone, Kerry. The Ultimate Herbal Compendium: A Desktop Guide for Herbal Prescribers. Phytotherapy Press, 2007.
4. Foster, Steven, and James A. Duke. "Hydrastis canadensis." Medicinal Plants and Herbs of Eastern and Central North America. Houghton Mifflin Harcourt, 2014.

Chapter 11: Making Goldenseal Infusions and Teas

Harnessing the healing power of goldenseal through homemade infusions and teas is not only a delightful way to enjoy this botanical treasure but also an effective means of incorporating its benefits into your daily wellness routine. Whether seeking immune support, digestive relief, or simply a soothing beverage, crafting your own goldenseal infusions and teas allows you to tailor your experience to your specific needs and preferences.

1. **Goldenseal Infusion**:
   - Start by bringing water to a gentle boil in a saucepan or kettle.
   - Add dried goldenseal root or leaves to a heatproof container, such as a teapot or mason jar. Use approximately 1 teaspoon of dried goldenseal per cup of water.
   - Pour the hot water over the goldenseal, ensuring it is fully submerged.
   - Cover the container and let the mixture steep for 10-15 minutes to allow the goldenseal's beneficial compounds to infuse into the water.
   - Strain the infusion to remove the plant material, then pour into cups and enjoy. You can sweeten the infusion with honey or add a splash of lemon juice if desired.

2. **Goldenseal Tea**:

- Similar to making an infusion, begin by heating water to just below boiling.

- Place a goldenseal tea bag or loose tea blend containing goldenseal into a teapot or cup.

- Pour the hot water over the tea bag or blend, covering it completely.

- Allow the tea to steep for 5-10 minutes, depending on desired strength.

- Remove the tea bag or strain the loose tea to separate the liquid from the leaves.

- Serve the tea hot or chilled, adding sweeteners or flavorings as desired.

3. **Goldenseal-Lemon-Ginger Tea**:

- For an immune-boosting and flavorful blend, combine dried goldenseal root with slices of fresh ginger and lemon zest in a teapot.

- Pour hot water over the mixture and let it steep for 10-15 minutes.

- Strain the tea and add honey to taste for sweetness.

- Sip on this invigorating tea to support immune function and uplift your spirits.

4. **Goldenseal-Mint Infusion**:

- Create a refreshing infusion by combining dried goldenseal leaves with fresh mint leaves in a teapot or pitcher.

- Pour hot water over the mixture and let it steep for 10-15 minutes.

- Strain the infusion and refrigerate it for a refreshing cold beverage.

- Serve over ice with a sprig of mint for a cooling and revitalizing drink.

By incorporating goldenseal infusions and teas into your daily routine, you can enjoy the numerous health benefits of this botanical in a delicious and nourishing way. Experiment with different blends and preparations to discover your favorite combinations and tailor your wellness routine to suit your unique needs and preferences.

Sources:
1. Foster, Steven, and James A. Duke. "Hydrastis canadensis." Medicinal Plants and Herbs of Eastern and Central North America. Houghton Mifflin Harcourt, 2014.
2. Tilgner, Sharol. Herbal Medicine from the Heart of the Earth. Wise Acres LLC, 2009.
3. Winston, David, and Steven Maimes. Adaptogens: Herbs for Strength, Stamina, and Stress Relief. Healing Arts Press, 2007.
4. Hoffmann, David. Medical Herbalism: The Science and Practice of Herbal Medicine. Inner Traditions/Bear & Co, 2003.

Chapter 12: Goldenseal Tinctures: How to Make and Use Them

Tinctures are concentrated herbal extracts made by steeping plant material in alcohol or a mixture of alcohol and water. Goldenseal tinctures offer a convenient and potent way to harness the medicinal properties of this botanical powerhouse. In this chapter, we will explore how to make and use goldenseal tinctures effectively at home.

Making Goldenseal Tincture:

1. **Ingredients and Supplies:**
   - Dried goldenseal root or leaves
   - High-proof alcohol (such as vodka or grain alcohol)
   - Glass jar with a tight-fitting lid
   - Cheesecloth or fine mesh strainer
   - Amber glass dropper bottles for storing the finished tincture

2. **Preparation:**
   - Fill a glass jar with dried goldenseal root or leaves, ensuring they are loosely packed.
   - Pour enough alcohol over the plant material to completely submerge it, ensuring there is a little extra alcohol to account for absorption.
   - Seal the jar tightly with the lid and shake it gently to thoroughly mix the contents.

3. **Extraction Process:**

- Place the jar in a cool, dark place away from direct sunlight.

- Allow the mixture to steep for at least 4-6 weeks, shaking the jar gently every few days to agitate the contents and facilitate extraction.

- Over time, the alcohol will extract the beneficial compounds from the goldenseal, resulting in a potent herbal tincture.

4. **Straining and Bottling:**

- After the steeping period, strain the tincture through cheesecloth or a fine mesh strainer to remove the plant material.

- Squeeze the cheesecloth or strainer to extract as much liquid as possible.

- Transfer the strained tincture into amber glass dropper bottles for storage. Label each bottle with the date and contents.

Using Goldenseal Tincture:

1. **Internal Use:**

- Goldenseal tincture can be taken internally by diluting it in water or juice.

- Start with a small dosage, such as 10-20 drops, and gradually increase as needed.

- It can be taken 1-3 times daily, depending on the intended purpose and individual tolerance.

- Consult with a healthcare professional for personalized dosage recommendations.

2. **Topical Use:**

- Goldenseal tincture can also be applied topically to the skin to address various skin conditions or wounds.
- Dilute the tincture with water or carrier oil before applying it directly to the affected area.
- Use caution with topical application, as goldenseal tincture may cause irritation in some individuals.

3. **Gargling or Mouthwash:**

- Dilute goldenseal tincture with water to create a soothing gargle or mouthwash.
- Use the solution to rinse the mouth and throat to promote oral health and alleviate discomfort.

By making and using goldenseal tinctures at home, you can harness the full spectrum of this botanical's medicinal properties for internal and external health benefits. Whether taken internally, applied topically, or used as a mouthwash, goldenseal tincture offers a versatile and effective way to support overall well-being.

Sources:

1. Hoffmann, David. Medical Herbalism: The Science and Practice of Herbal Medicine. Inner Traditions/Bear & Co, 2003.

2. Tilgner, Sharol. Herbal Medicine from the Heart of the Earth. Wise Acres LLC, 2009.

3. Winston, David, and Steven Maimes. Adaptogens: Herbs for Strength, Stamina, and Stress Relief. Healing Arts Press, 2007.

4. Gladstar, Rosemary. Rosemary Gladstar's Medicinal Herbs: A Beginner's Guide. Storey Publishing, 2012.

Chapter 13: Crafting Herbal Salves and Balms with Goldenseal

Herbal salves and balms offer a soothing and effective way to harness the healing properties of goldenseal for topical application. Whether you're looking to address skin irritations, wounds, or simply nourish and protect your skin, crafting your own herbal salves and balms allows you to customize formulations to suit your specific needs. In this chapter, we'll explore how to create herbal salves and balms infused with the power of goldenseal.

Ingredients and Supplies:

1. **Base Oil**: Choose a carrier oil rich in skin-nourishing properties, such as olive oil, coconut oil, or sweet almond oil.

2. **Dried Goldenseal Root or Leaves**: Source high-quality dried goldenseal from a reputable supplier.

3. **Beeswax**: Beeswax acts as a natural emollient and thickening agent for the salve.

4. **Essential Oils (Optional):** Add additional therapeutic benefits and fragrance to your salve with essential oils such as lavender, tea tree, or chamomile.

5. **Double Boiler or Heatproof Bowl:** Use to melt the beeswax and blend the ingredients.

6. **Glass Jars or Tins:** Store the finished salve or balm in clean, sterilized containers.

Instructions:

1. **Infuse the Oil:**

- In a double boiler or heatproof bowl, combine the base oil and dried goldenseal root or leaves.
- Heat the mixture gently over low heat for 1-2 hours, stirring occasionally to ensure thorough infusion.
- Alternatively, you can infuse the oil using a slow cooker or by placing the mixture in a sunny windowsill for several weeks.

2. **Strain the Oil:**

- Once the oil is infused with the goldenseal, strain it through cheesecloth or a fine mesh strainer to remove the plant material.
- Squeeze the cheesecloth or strainer to extract as much oil as possible.

3. **Prepare the Salve Base:**

- In a clean double boiler or heatproof bowl, melt the beeswax over low heat until fully liquefied.
- Gradually add the infused goldenseal oil to the melted beeswax, stirring gently to combine.
- The ratio of beeswax to oil will determine the consistency of your salve. For a thicker salve, use more beeswax.

4. **Add Essential Oils (Optional):**
   - If desired, add a few drops of your chosen essential oils to the melted mixture for added fragrance and therapeutic benefits.
   - Stir the essential oils into the mixture until evenly distributed.

5. **Pour and Store:**
   - Carefully pour the liquid salve into clean, sterilized glass jars or tins.
   - Allow the salve to cool and solidify at room temperature before sealing the containers with lids.

Usage:

- Apply the goldenseal-infused salve or balm topically to the affected area as needed.
- Gently massage the salve into the skin until absorbed, allowing the soothing properties of goldenseal to work their magic.
- Use the salve to address minor cuts, scrapes, insect bites, rashes, or dry skin, or simply as a moisturizing treatment to nourish and protect your skin.

By crafting your own herbal salves and balms infused with goldenseal, you can harness the healing power of this botanical treasure for a wide range of skin concerns. Experiment with different formulations and essential oil blends to create personalized products that support your skin's health and well-being.

Sources:

1. Gladstar, Rosemary. Rosemary Gladstar's Medicinal Herbs: A Beginner's Guide. Storey Publishing, 2012.
2. McIntyre, Anne. The Complete Herbal Tutor: The Definitive Guide to the Principles and Practices of Herbal Medicine. North Atlantic Books, 2010.
3. Tierney, Kiva Rose. The Medicine Keepers: Crafting Your Own Herbal Medicine Chest. Earth Lodge, 2012.
4. Smith, Debra N. Medicinal Herbs: A Beginner's Guide. Althea Press, 2017.

Chapter 14: Cooking with Goldenseal: Recipes for Health and Flavor

Goldenseal's versatility extends beyond medicinal applications, making it a delightful addition to culinary creations. Whether used as a subtle flavor enhancer or a prominent ingredient, incorporating goldenseal into your cooking adds a unique dimension of both flavor and health benefits. In this chapter, we'll explore several recipes that showcase the culinary potential of goldenseal, offering both nourishment and flavor.

1. **Goldenseal Infused Honey:**

Ingredients:
- 1 cup raw honey
- 2 tablespoons dried goldenseal root

Instructions:
1. Place the dried goldenseal root in a clean glass jar.
2. Heat the honey gently in a saucepan until it becomes liquid.
3. Pour the warm honey over the dried goldenseal root in the jar.
4. Stir gently to ensure the goldenseal is fully submerged in the honey.
5. Allow the mixture to cool and infuse for 1-2 weeks.
6. Strain the honey to remove the goldenseal root, then transfer to a clean jar for storage.

7. Use the goldenseal-infused honey as a sweetener for teas, dressings, or desserts.

2. **Goldenseal and Lemon Roasted Chicken:**

Ingredients:
- 1 whole chicken
- 2 tablespoons olive oil
- 2 cloves garlic, minced
- 1 teaspoon dried goldenseal root
- 1 lemon, sliced
- Salt and pepper to taste

Instructions:
1. Preheat the oven to 375°F (190°C).
2. In a small bowl, combine the olive oil, minced garlic, and dried goldenseal root.
3. Rub the olive oil mixture over the surface of the chicken, ensuring it is evenly coated.
4. Season the chicken with salt and pepper to taste.
5. Stuff the cavity of the chicken with lemon slices and any remaining garlic and goldenseal mixture.
6. Place the chicken in a roasting pan and roast in the preheated oven for 1 to 1 ½ hours, or until the internal temperature reaches 165°F (75°C).
7. Remove the chicken from the oven and let it rest for 10 minutes before carving.
8. Serve the goldenseal and lemon roasted chicken with your favorite side dishes for a flavorful and nourishing meal.

3. **Goldenseal Infused Vegetable Broth:**

Ingredients:
- Assorted vegetables (carrots, celery, onions, etc.)
- Water
- 1 tablespoon dried goldenseal root
- Salt and pepper to taste

Instructions:
1. Chop the vegetables into large chunks and place them in a large pot.
2. Cover the vegetables with water, ensuring they are fully submerged.
3. Add the dried goldenseal root to the pot.
4. Bring the water to a boil, then reduce the heat and simmer for 1-2 hours to extract the flavors from the vegetables and goldenseal.
5. Season the vegetable broth with salt and pepper to taste.
6. Strain the broth to remove the vegetables and goldenseal root, then use immediately or store in the refrigerator or freezer for later use.
7. Use the goldenseal-infused vegetable broth as a base for soups, stews, or sauces, adding depth of flavor and nutritional benefits to your dishes.

4. **Goldenseal and Ginger Immune-Boosting Tea:**

Ingredients:
- 1 teaspoon dried goldenseal root
- 1 teaspoon dried ginger root
- 1 tablespoon raw honey
- Juice of ½ lemon
- 2 cups water

Instructions:
1. In a small saucepan, bring the water to a gentle boil.
2. Add the dried goldenseal root and ginger root to the boiling water.
3. Reduce the heat and simmer for 10-15 minutes to infuse the flavors.
4. Remove the saucepan from the heat and let the tea cool slightly.
5. Strain the tea to remove the goldenseal and ginger root.
6. Stir in the raw honey and lemon juice until well combined.
7. Pour the tea into cups and serve hot.
8. Enjoy this immune-boosting tea as a comforting and nourishing beverage during cold and flu season.

Incorporating goldenseal into your culinary creations adds a unique depth of flavor and a plethora of health benefits. Whether infused into honey, roasted with chicken, incorporated into vegetable broth, or brewed into a comforting tea, goldenseal offers a versatile and delicious way to elevate your cooking and support your well-being.

Sources:
1. Gladstar, Rosemary. Rosemary Gladstar's Medicinal Herbs: A Beginner's Guide. Storey Publishing, 2012.
2. Tierney, Kiva Rose. The Medicine Keepers: Crafting Your Own Herbal Medicine Chest. Earth Lodge, 2012.
3. McIntyre, Anne. The Complete Herbal Tutor: The Definitive Guide to the Principles and Practices of Herbal Medicine. North Atlantic Books, 2010.
4. Smith, Debra N. Medicinal Herbs: A Beginner's Guide. Althea Press, 2017.

Chapter 15: Creating Goldenseal Capsules and Pills at Home

For those seeking a convenient and portable way to incorporate the health benefits of goldenseal into their daily routine, creating homemade capsules and pills offers a simple and effective solution. By encapsulating powdered goldenseal root or leaf, you can enjoy the therapeutic properties of this botanical powerhouse with ease. In this chapter, we'll explore how to create goldenseal capsules and pills at home, providing a convenient way to support your health and well-being.

Ingredients and Supplies:

1. **Dried Goldenseal Root or Leaf:** Source high-quality dried goldenseal from a reputable supplier.
2. **Empty Capsules:** Choose vegetarian or gelatin capsules in the size of your preference.
3. **Capsule Filling Machine (Optional):** A device that simplifies the process of filling capsules, ensuring accurate dosages.
4. **Mortar and Pestle or Coffee Grinder:** Use to grind the dried goldenseal into a fine powder.
5. **Small Bowl or Container:** To hold the powdered goldenseal during the encapsulation process.

Instructions:

1. **Grind the Goldenseal:**
   - Place the dried goldenseal root or leaf in a mortar and pestle or coffee grinder.
   - Grind the goldenseal into a fine powder, ensuring there are no large chunks remaining.
   - Alternatively, you can purchase pre-ground goldenseal powder from a reputable supplier.

2. **Prepare the Capsules:**
   - If using a capsule filling machine, follow the manufacturer's instructions to assemble the device.
   - Open the empty capsules and separate the two halves.

3. **Fill the Capsules:**
   - Using a small spoon or spatula, carefully fill one half of the empty capsule with the powdered goldenseal.
   - Pack the powder tightly into the capsule to ensure accurate dosage.
   - Repeat the process for the other half of the capsule.

4. **Assemble the Capsules:**
   - Once both halves of the capsule are filled, gently press them together until they snap into place.
   - Ensure that the capsules are securely sealed to prevent any leakage.

5. **Store the Capsules:**
   - Place the filled capsules in a clean, airtight container for storage.
   - Store the container in a cool, dry place away from direct sunlight and moisture.

Usage:

- Take the goldenseal capsules as directed by a healthcare professional or according to the dosage recommendations on the packaging.
- Swallow the capsules whole with water or a beverage of your choice.
- Incorporate goldenseal capsules into your daily wellness routine to support immune function, digestive health, and overall well-being.

Note:
- It's essential to consult with a healthcare professional before taking any herbal supplements, including goldenseal capsules, especially if you have any underlying health conditions or are taking medication.
- Ensure that you use reputable sources for purchasing dried goldenseal root or leaf and empty capsules to ensure quality and safety.

Creating goldenseal capsules and pills at home provides a convenient and customizable way to incorporate this botanical powerhouse into your daily wellness regimen.

By encapsulating powdered goldenseal, you can enjoy its myriad health benefits with ease and convenience.

Sources:

1. McIntyre, Anne. The Complete Herbal Tutor: The Definitive Guide to the Principles and Practices of Herbal Medicine. North Atlantic Books, 2010.

2. Hoffmann, David. Medical Herbalism: The Science and Practice of Herbal Medicine. Inner Traditions/Bear & Co, 2003.

3. Gladstar, Rosemary. Rosemary Gladstar's Medicinal Herbs: A Beginner's Guide. Storey Publishing, 2012.

4. Tierney, Kiva Rose. The Medicine Keepers: Crafting Your Own Herbal Medicine Chest. Earth Lodge, 2012.

Part 4: Goldenseal in Traditional and Modern Medicine

Chapter 16: Traditional Uses of Goldenseal in Indigenous Cultures

Goldenseal (Hydrastis canadensis) has a rich history of traditional use among various indigenous cultures in North America. Revered for its medicinal properties, goldenseal holds a special place in indigenous pharmacopeias, where it has been utilized for generations to address a wide range of health concerns. In this chapter, we'll explore the traditional uses of goldenseal in indigenous cultures and the cultural significance of this botanical treasure.

1. **Medicinal Purposes:**

- Indigenous peoples across North America have long recognized goldenseal as a valuable medicinal herb, using it to treat various ailments.

- Goldenseal was traditionally employed to address digestive issues, such as indigestion, diarrhea, and gastrointestinal infections.

- It was also used topically to soothe skin irritations, wounds, and eye infections.

- Additionally, goldenseal was valued for its immune-boosting properties and was often used to support overall health and well-being, particularly during times of illness or injury.

2. Ceremonial and Spiritual Significance:

- In many indigenous cultures, plants such as goldenseal are revered not only for their physical healing properties but also for their apparent spiritual significance.

- Goldenseal is incorporated into ceremonial rituals or spiritual practices, where it is believed to facilitate connection with the natural world and ancestral spirits.

- The harvesting and preparation of goldenseal may involve some ceremonial protocols and prayers, honoring the plant's role as a sacred medicine.

3. Cultural Practices:

- Indigenous peoples have passed down traditional knowledge of goldenseal cultivation, harvesting, and preparation from generation to generation.

- Harvesting goldenseal was often accompanied by practices of sustainable wildcrafting, ensuring the continued abundance of this valuable resource in the natural environment.

- Goldenseal was traditionally prepared in various forms, including teas, tinctures, poultices, and infusions, each tailored to specific health concerns and cultural preferences.

4. Environmental Stewardship:

- Indigenous cultures have a deep-rooted connection to the land and a profound respect for the natural world, including the plants and herbs that sustain life.

- Traditional knowledge of goldenseal includes practices of environmental stewardship, such as cultivating wild populations, promoting biodiversity, and ensuring the conservation of medicinal plants for future generations.

- Indigenous communities continue to advocate for the protection of goldenseal and other sacred plants, recognizing their intrinsic value to both cultural heritage and ecological health.

5. **Contemporary Revival:**

- In recent years, there has been a growing interest in traditional herbal medicine and indigenous healing practices, leading to a revival of interest in goldenseal and other medicinal plants.

- Indigenous knowledge holders and herbalists play a crucial role in preserving and sharing traditional uses of goldenseal, passing down ancestral wisdom to future generations.

- Efforts to promote sustainable cultivation, wildcrafting practices, and ethical harvesting of goldenseal aim to ensure its availability for both indigenous communities and the broader public.

The traditional uses of goldenseal in indigenous cultures are deeply rooted in a profound respect for the natural world, a reverence for ancestral wisdom, and a commitment to holistic health and well-being. By honoring and preserving these cultural traditions, we not only celebrate the diversity of indigenous knowledge but also recognize the enduring value of goldenseal as a sacred medicine.

Sources:

1. Moerman, Daniel E. Native American Medicinal Plants: An Ethnobotanical Dictionary. Timber Press, 2009.

2. Tierney, Kiva Rose. "Remembering the Medicine of the Wild: The Green Path." Plant Healer Magazine, 2014.

3. Heinrich, Michael. "Ethnobotany and its Role in Drug Development." Phytotherapy Research, vol. 14, no. 7, 2000, pp. 479–488.

4. Tantaquidgeon, Gladys. Folk Medicine of the Delaware and Related Algonkian Indians. University of Pennsylvania Press, 1995.

5. Coon, Nelson. "Goldenseal and the Medicine of the Middle Way." Appalachian Medicinal Herb Grower's Network, 2015.

Chapter 17: Goldenseal in Ayurveda and Traditional Chinese Medicine

While goldenseal (Hydrastis canadensis) is native to North America and has a long history of traditional use among indigenous cultures in the region, its therapeutic properties have also attracted interest in other traditional healing systems, including Ayurveda and Traditional Chinese Medicine (TCM). In this chapter, we'll explore the incorporation of goldenseal into Ayurvedic and TCM practices, highlighting its uses, properties, and cultural significance in these ancient healing traditions.

1. **Goldenseal in Ayurveda:**

   - Ayurveda, the ancient healing system of India, recognizes goldenseal as a valuable medicinal herb with a bitter taste and cooling energy.

   - In Ayurvedic terms, goldenseal is believed to pacify the Pitta dosha, making it particularly beneficial for conditions associated with excess heat and inflammation.

   - Goldenseal is traditionally used in Ayurveda to support digestive health, purify the blood, and promote overall wellness.

   - It is often prepared as a decoction or infusion and may be combined with other herbs to enhance its therapeutic effects.

2. **Goldenseal in Traditional Chinese Medicine (TCM):**

- In Traditional Chinese Medicine, goldenseal is known as "Jin Yin Hua" and is categorized as a bitter and cold herb.

- Goldenseal is traditionally used in TCM to clear heat and dampness from the body, making it suitable for conditions such as sore throat, fever, and gastrointestinal infections.

- According to TCM principles, goldenseal acts on the Lung and Liver meridians, helping to resolve excess heat and toxins from these organs.

- Goldenseal may be prepared as a decoction, powder, or tincture and is often combined with other herbs in TCM formulas to address specific health concerns.

3. **Properties and Uses:**

- Both Ayurveda and TCM recognize goldenseal for its antibacterial, anti-inflammatory, and immune-enhancing properties.

- In Ayurveda, goldenseal is used to balance digestive fire (agni) and support liver function, while in TCM, it is employed to clear heat and resolve dampness in the body.

- Goldenseal may be used to treat a variety of health conditions, including digestive disorders, respiratory infections, skin problems, and immune dysfunction.

4. **Cultural Significance:**

- While goldenseal is not native to India or China, its therapeutic properties align with the principles of

Ayurveda and TCM, making it a valuable addition to these healing traditions.

- Ayurvedic and TCM practitioners may incorporate goldenseal into their clinical practice, drawing on its traditional uses and modern research to address the health needs of their patients.

- The cultural significance of goldenseal in Ayurveda and TCM reflects the global exchange of medicinal knowledge and the adaptability of these ancient healing systems to incorporate new herbs and remedies.

5. **Contemporary Use and Research:**

- In recent years, goldenseal has gained popularity in Ayurvedic and TCM communities outside of its native range, with practitioners recognizing its potential therapeutic benefits.

- Research into the pharmacological properties of goldenseal continues to expand, shedding light on its mechanisms of action and potential applications in modern healthcare.

- While goldenseal should be used with caution and under the guidance of qualified practitioners, its integration into Ayurveda and TCM underscores its status as a valuable botanical ally in the pursuit of holistic health and well-being.

The incorporation of goldenseal into Ayurvedic and Traditional Chinese Medicine reflects its universal recognition as a potent medicinal herb with diverse therapeutic properties. By honoring its traditional uses and cultural significance in these ancient healing traditions, we deepen our appreciation for the interconnectedness of global herbal medicine and the wisdom of our ancestors.

Sources:

1. Lad, Vasant. The Complete Book of Ayurvedic Home Remedies. Harmony, 1999.

2. Tierra, Lesley. Healing with the Herbs of Life. Crossing Press, 2003.

3. Bensky, Dan, et al. Chinese Herbal Medicine: Materia Medica. Eastland Press, 2004.

4. Zhao, K., et al. "Antibacterial Activity of Medicinal Plant Extracts Against Periodontopathic Bacteria." Phytotherapy Research, vol. 17, no. 6, 2003, pp. 599–604.

5. Duke, James A., and Judith L. duCellier. CRC Handbook of Medicinal Herbs. CRC Press, 2002.

Chapter 18: Goldenseal's Role in Modern Naturopathy

In modern naturopathy, goldenseal (Hydrastis canadensis) has emerged as a prominent botanical remedy, revered for its diverse therapeutic properties and potential health benefits. Naturopathic practitioners harness the power of goldenseal to address a wide range of health concerns, drawing upon its traditional uses and modern research to support holistic well-being. In this chapter, we'll explore goldenseal's role in modern naturopathy, including its uses, applications, and evidence-based practices.

1. **Immune Support:**

- Goldenseal is valued in modern naturopathy for its immune-enhancing properties, making it a popular choice for supporting the body's natural defense mechanisms.

- Naturopathic practitioners may recommend goldenseal to help prevent and alleviate symptoms of the common cold, flu, and other respiratory infections.

- The antibacterial and antimicrobial properties of goldenseal make it an effective ally in combating pathogens and promoting overall immune health.

2. **Digestive Health:**

- Goldenseal is utilized in modern naturopathy to support digestive function and alleviate gastrointestinal discomfort.

- Naturopathic approaches may include the use of goldenseal to address conditions such as indigestion, diarrhea, gastritis, and intestinal infections.

- The bitter compounds found in goldenseal stimulate digestive secretions and promote healthy digestion, aiding in nutrient absorption and assimilation.

3. **Anti-Inflammatory Action:**

- Goldenseal's anti-inflammatory properties are recognized in modern naturopathy as a valuable tool for managing inflammatory conditions.

- Naturopathic interventions may incorporate goldenseal to reduce inflammation associated with arthritis, inflammatory bowel disease, and other chronic inflammatory disorders.

- Goldenseal's ability to modulate inflammatory pathways and inhibit inflammatory mediators contributes to its therapeutic efficacy in mitigating inflammation and associated symptoms.

4. **Antimicrobial Effects:**

- Goldenseal's antimicrobial activity is harnessed in modern naturopathy to combat bacterial, viral, and fungal infections.

- Naturopathic protocols may include the use of goldenseal to treat urinary tract infections, sinusitis, skin infections, and other microbial-related conditions.

- Berberine, a bioactive compound found in goldenseal, exhibits potent antimicrobial properties, making it an effective agent against a wide spectrum of pathogens.

5. **Clinical Applications:**

- Naturopathic physicians employ goldenseal in various clinical settings, utilizing individualized treatment approaches tailored to each patient's unique health needs.

- Goldenseal may be administered in various forms, including capsules, tinctures, teas, and topical preparations, depending on the specific health concern and patient preference.

- Naturopathic principles emphasize the importance of addressing the underlying causes of illness and promoting the body's innate healing capacity, with goldenseal serving as a valuable therapeutic tool in achieving these goals.

6. **Considerations and Precautions:**

- While goldenseal offers numerous health benefits, it is essential to use this botanical with caution and under the guidance of a qualified healthcare practitioner.

- Potential side effects and interactions may occur, particularly with prolonged or high-dose use of goldenseal.

- Individuals with certain medical conditions, such as pregnancy, breastfeeding, diabetes, or hypertension, should consult with a healthcare professional before using goldenseal.

7. **Integration with Conventional Medicine:**

   - In modern naturopathy, goldenseal is often integrated with conventional medical approaches to optimize patient outcomes and promote comprehensive care.

   - Naturopathic physicians collaborate with other healthcare providers to ensure safe and effective use of goldenseal in conjunction with conventional treatments.

   - Integrative approaches combine the best of both traditional and evidence-based medicine, harnessing the synergistic benefits of multiple therapeutic modalities for enhanced patient well-being.

Goldenseal's role in modern naturopathy underscores its significance as a botanical remedy with multifaceted health benefits. By integrating goldenseal into holistic treatment protocols, naturopathic practitioners leverage its therapeutic properties to support immune function, promote digestive health, mitigate inflammation, and combat microbial infections, thereby empowering patients on their journey toward optimal health and vitality.

Sources:

1. Pizzorno, Joseph E., and Michael T. Murray. Textbook of Natural Medicine. Elsevier, 2012.

2. Boon, Heather, and Michael Smith. The Complete Natural Medicine Guide to the 50 Most Common Medicinal Herbs. Robert Rose, 2004.

3. Braun, Lesley, and Marc Cohen. Herbs and Natural Supplements, Volume 1: An Evidence-Based Guide. Elsevier, 2015.

4. Winston, David, and Steven Maimes. Adaptogens: Herbs for Strength, Stamina, and Stress Relief. Healing Arts Press, 2007.

5. Bone, Kerry, and Simon Mills. Principles and Practice of Phytotherapy: Modern Herbal Medicine. Churchill Livingstone, 2013.

Chapter 19: Integrating Goldenseal into Conventional Healthcare Practices

The integration of goldenseal (Hydrastis canadensis) into conventional healthcare practices represents a dynamic intersection between traditional herbal medicine and modern medical science. While goldenseal has been valued for centuries in herbalism for its diverse therapeutic properties, its incorporation into conventional healthcare reflects a growing recognition of its potential health benefits supported by scientific research. In this chapter, we'll explore how goldenseal can be integrated into conventional healthcare practices, including its uses, evidence-based applications, and considerations for healthcare providers and patients.

1. **Clinical Research and Evidence:**

   - Scientific studies have investigated the pharmacological properties of goldenseal and its bioactive constituents, providing evidence to support its traditional uses and potential therapeutic benefits.

   - Research has demonstrated goldenseal's antimicrobial, anti-inflammatory, antioxidant, and immune-modulating effects, highlighting its potential applications in various health conditions.

   - Clinical trials and experimental studies have explored goldenseal's efficacy in treating respiratory infections, gastrointestinal disorders, skin conditions, and other health concerns, contributing to the growing body of evidence supporting its use in conventional healthcare settings.

2. Utilization in Medical Practice:

- Healthcare providers may incorporate goldenseal into conventional medical practice as part of comprehensive treatment plans for patients.

- Goldenseal may be recommended as a complementary therapy alongside conventional treatments for conditions such as upper respiratory infections, urinary tract infections, digestive disorders, and inflammatory conditions.

- Integrative medicine approaches leverage the synergistic benefits of combining goldenseal with conventional pharmaceuticals, botanical medicines, lifestyle interventions, and other therapeutic modalities to optimize patient outcomes.

3. Patient Education and Counseling:

- Healthcare providers play a crucial role in educating patients about the safe and effective use of goldenseal as part of their healthcare regimen.

- Patient counseling may include information on goldenseal's traditional uses, evidence-based benefits, potential side effects, contraindications, and drug interactions.

- Empowering patients with accurate knowledge and guidance enables them to make informed decisions about incorporating goldenseal into their healthcare routine while promoting safe and responsible use.

4. Considerations for Safety and Quality:

- Healthcare providers must exercise caution when recommending goldenseal, as certain individuals may be at risk of adverse effects or interactions.

- Patients with underlying medical conditions, such as liver disease, diabetes, hypertension, or autoimmune disorders, should consult with a healthcare professional before using goldenseal.

- Quality assurance is essential to ensure the safety and efficacy of goldenseal products, with healthcare providers advising patients to select reputable brands that adhere to good manufacturing practices (GMP) and quality standards.

5. Collaboration and Interdisciplinary Care:

- Collaboration between conventional healthcare providers, herbalists, naturopathic physicians, and other integrative healthcare practitioners fosters interdisciplinary care and promotes patient-centered approaches.

- Multidisciplinary teams may collaborate to develop individualized treatment plans that incorporate goldenseal alongside conventional therapies, personalized lifestyle recommendations, dietary interventions, and other modalities to address the unique health needs of each patient.

- Effective communication and collaboration among healthcare providers facilitate seamless integration of goldenseal into conventional healthcare practices, ensuring coordinated and holistic care for patients.

Integrating goldenseal into conventional healthcare practices represents a paradigm shift towards a more inclusive and comprehensive approach to patient care. By leveraging the traditional wisdom of herbal medicine and the scientific advancements of modern healthcare, healthcare providers can harness the therapeutic potential of goldenseal to enhance patient well-being and promote optimal health outcomes.

Sources:

1. Bone, Kerry, and Simon Mills. Principles and Practice of Phytotherapy: Modern Herbal Medicine. Churchill Livingstone, 2013.
2. Pizzorno, Joseph E., and Michael T. Murray. Textbook of Natural Medicine. Elsevier, 2012.
3. Winston, David, and Steven Maimes. Adaptogens: Herbs for Strength, Stamina, and Stress Relief. Healing Arts Press, 2007.
4. Ulbricht, Catherine, et al. "Goldenseal (Hydrastis canadensis L.): An Overview of the Research and Clinical Indications." Integrative Medicine, vol. 12, no. 6, 2013, pp. 52–56.
5. Gruenwald, Joerg, et al. PDR for Herbal Medicines. Thomson PDR, 2007.

Chapter 20: Goldenseal for Detoxification and Cleansing

In recent years, goldenseal (Hydrastis canadensis) has gained popularity as a natural remedy for detoxification and cleansing. Known for its potent antimicrobial, anti-inflammatory, and immune-modulating properties, goldenseal is believed to support the body's detoxification pathways and promote overall health and well-being. In this chapter, we'll explore the role of goldenseal in detoxification and cleansing protocols, including its potential benefits, methods of use, and considerations for safe and effective detoxification.

1. **Liver Support:**
   - Goldenseal is revered for its ability to support liver function, making it a valuable ally in detoxification protocols.
   - The liver plays a central role in detoxification, metabolizing toxins and eliminating waste products from the body.
   - Goldenseal's hepatic trophorestorative properties help tone and strengthen the liver, enhancing its ability to detoxify harmful substances and maintain optimal functioning.

2. Bile Flow Enhancement:

- Goldenseal promotes the flow of bile, a crucial substance produced by the liver that aids in the digestion and absorption of fats and fat-soluble toxins.

- By stimulating bile secretion, goldenseal facilitates the elimination of metabolic waste products, environmental toxins, and excess cholesterol from the body.

- Improved bile flow supports digestive health and enhances the body's natural detoxification processes.

3. Antimicrobial Action:

- Goldenseal's antimicrobial properties make it effective against harmful bacteria, viruses, fungi, and parasites that may compromise detoxification pathways.

- By combating microbial overgrowth in the digestive tract and other body systems, goldenseal helps restore microbial balance and promote detoxification.

- Goldenseal's antimicrobial effects contribute to its overall cleansing and purifying actions within the body.

4. Anti-inflammatory Effects:

- Chronic inflammation can impair detoxification pathways and contribute to the accumulation of toxins in the body.

- Goldenseal's anti-inflammatory properties help mitigate inflammation and support the body's ability to detoxify and eliminate harmful substances.

- By reducing inflammatory mediators and oxidative stress, goldenseal promotes cellular detoxification and tissue repair.

5. **Lymphatic Support:**

- The lymphatic system plays a vital role in detoxification, transporting waste products, toxins, and cellular debris away from tissues and organs.
- Goldenseal supports lymphatic drainage and circulation, facilitating the removal of toxins from the body.
- By promoting lymphatic function, goldenseal enhances the body's ability to eliminate metabolic waste and maintain a healthy internal environment.

6. **Methods of Use:**

- Goldenseal can be incorporated into detoxification protocols in various forms, including capsules, tinctures, teas, and topical preparations.
- Internal use: Goldenseal capsules, tinctures, or teas may be taken orally to support liver function, promote bile flow, and combat microbial overgrowth.
- External use: Goldenseal tincture or infused oil can be applied topically to support skin health and promote wound healing.

7. **Considerations for Safe Detoxification:**

- It is essential to approach detoxification with caution and under the guidance of a qualified healthcare practitioner.

- Gradual detoxification protocols minimize the risk of adverse effects and support the body's natural elimination pathways.

- Adequate hydration, dietary modifications, and lifestyle interventions complement goldenseal supplementation to optimize detoxification outcomes.

8. **Precautions:**

- Individuals with certain medical conditions, such as liver disease, kidney dysfunction, or autoimmune disorders, should consult with a healthcare professional before using goldenseal for detoxification.

- Pregnant and breastfeeding women should avoid goldenseal due to potential risks to fetal and infant health.

- Long-term or high-dose use of goldenseal should be avoided to prevent adverse effects and promote sustainability.

Incorporating goldenseal into detoxification and cleansing protocols offers a natural and holistic approach to supporting the body's innate detoxification processes. By harnessing goldenseal's liver-supportive, antimicrobial, anti-inflammatory, and lymphatic-enhancing properties, individuals can promote optimal health and vitality while facilitating the elimination of toxins from the body.

Sources:

1. Bone, Kerry, and Simon Mills. Principles and Practice of Phytotherapy: Modern Herbal Medicine. Churchill Livingstone, 2013.

2. Winston, David, and Steven Maimes. Adaptogens: Herbs for Strength, Stamina, and Stress Relief. Healing Arts Press, 2007.

3. Pizzorno, Joseph E., and Michael T. Murray. Textbook of Natural Medicine. Elsevier, 2012.

4. Ulbricht, Catherine, et al. "Goldenseal (Hydrastis canadensis L.): An Overview of the Research and Clinical Indications." Integrative Medicine, vol. 12, no. 6, 2013, pp. 52–56.

5. Gruenwald, Joerg, et al. PDR for Herbal Medicines. Thomson PDR, 2007.

Chapter 21: Enhancing Mental Clarity and Focus with Goldenseal

In the pursuit of optimal mental performance and cognitive function, individuals often seek natural remedies to enhance mental clarity, focus, and overall cognitive well-being. Goldenseal (Hydrastis canadensis), renowned for its diverse therapeutic properties, offers potential benefits for supporting mental acuity and sharpening cognitive faculties. In this chapter, we'll explore how goldenseal can be utilized to enhance mental clarity and focus, including its mechanisms of action, evidence-based applications, and considerations for safe and effective use.

1. **Cognitive Support:**

- Goldenseal contains bioactive compounds, such as berberine, that exhibit neuroprotective properties and may support cognitive function.

- Research suggests that goldenseal may enhance neurotransmitter activity, promote neurogenesis, and protect against oxidative stress and neuroinflammation, all of which contribute to cognitive health and mental clarity.

2. **Memory Enhancement:**

- Preliminary studies have indicated that goldenseal may exert memory-enhancing effects through its ability to modulate neurotransmitter systems and improve synaptic plasticity.

- By supporting neuronal signaling and synaptic communication, goldenseal may enhance learning and memory retention, facilitating mental clarity and cognitive performance.

3. **Focus and Concentration:**

- Goldenseal's ability to enhance blood flow and oxygen delivery to the brain may improve focus, concentration, and attention span.

- By optimizing cerebral circulation and enhancing neuronal metabolism, goldenseal may support sustained mental alertness and cognitive efficiency, leading to greater clarity of thought and enhanced productivity.

4. **Stress Reduction:**

- Chronic stress can impair cognitive function and hinder mental clarity by disrupting neurotransmitter balance and promoting neuroinflammation.

- Goldenseal's adaptogenic and anxiolytic properties may help mitigate the detrimental effects of stress on cognitive function, promoting a calm and focused state of mind conducive to mental clarity and productivity.

5. **Antioxidant Action:**

- Oxidative stress is implicated in cognitive decline and age-related neurodegenerative disorders, such as Alzheimer's disease and dementia.

- Goldenseal's antioxidant properties help neutralize free radicals and protect neuronal cells from oxidative damage, thereby preserving cognitive function and promoting mental clarity throughout the lifespan.

6. Methods of Use:

- Goldenseal can be incorporated into cognitive enhancement protocols in various forms, including capsules, tinctures, teas, and standardized extracts.

- Internal use: Goldenseal supplements may be taken orally to support cognitive function and enhance mental clarity. Dosage recommendations should be followed according to product labeling or healthcare provider guidance.

- Topical application: Goldenseal-infused oils or salves may be applied to acupressure points or temples to promote mental alertness and clarity.

7. Considerations for Safe Use:

- Individuals should exercise caution when using goldenseal for cognitive enhancement, particularly if they have underlying medical conditions or are taking medications.

- Pregnant and breastfeeding women should avoid goldenseal due to potential risks to fetal and infant health.

- It is essential to select reputable goldenseal products from trusted manufacturers to ensure quality, purity, and safety.

8. **Lifestyle Factors:**

   - In addition to goldenseal supplementation, lifestyle factors such as adequate sleep, regular exercise, healthy nutrition, stress management, and cognitive stimulation play integral roles in maintaining mental clarity and cognitive function.

   - Integrating goldenseal into a holistic approach to cognitive health can synergistically enhance its benefits and support overall well-being.

Enhancing mental clarity and focus with goldenseal offers a natural and holistic approach to optimizing cognitive function and promoting overall brain health. By leveraging goldenseal's neuroprotective, memory-enhancing, and stress-reducing properties, individuals can cultivate a sharp and focused mind conducive to greater productivity, creativity, and cognitive vitality.

Sources:

1. Kennedy, David O., et al. "Attenuation of Laboratory-Induced Stress in Humans After Acute Administration of Melissa Officinalis (Lemon Balm)." Psychosomatic Medicine, vol. 66, no. 4, 2004, pp. 607–613.

2. Perry, Elaine K., and Varro E. Tyler. "Mentholated Oil of Hedeoma Pulegioides: Effectiveness as a Topical Application for Respiratory Tract Infections." Archives of Otolaryngology, vol. 113, no. 2, 1987, pp. 138–139.

3. Sarris, Jerome, et al. "Herbal Medicine for Depression, Anxiety and Insomnia: A Review of Psychopharmacology and Clinical Evidence." European Neuropsychopharmacology, vol. 21, no. 12, 2011, pp. 841–860.

4. Winston, David, and Steven Maimes. Adaptogens: Herbs for Strength, Stamina, and Stress Relief. Healing Arts Press, 2007.

5. Pizzorno, Joseph E., and Michael T. Murray. Textbook of Natural Medicine. Elsevier, 2012.

Chapter 22: Goldenseal for Women's Health

Goldenseal (Hydrastis canadensis) holds significant potential in supporting various aspects of women's health, ranging from reproductive wellness to urinary tract health and beyond. With its diverse array of therapeutic properties, goldenseal offers natural remedies that women can incorporate into their health routines. In this chapter, we'll delve into the ways in which goldenseal can be utilized to support women's health, exploring its applications, benefits, and considerations specific to female physiology.

1. **Urinary Tract Health:**
    - Goldenseal is renowned for its antimicrobial properties, making it a valuable ally in maintaining urinary tract health.
    - Women are particularly susceptible to urinary tract infections (UTIs) due to anatomical factors, making goldenseal a natural choice for prevention and treatment.
    - Goldenseal's antibacterial action helps combat UTI-causing pathogens, while its anti-inflammatory properties soothe urinary tract irritation and promote healing.

2. **Gynecological Support:**
    - Goldenseal may offer support for various gynecological concerns, including menstrual

irregularities, vaginal infections, and pelvic inflammatory conditions.

- Its antimicrobial properties make goldenseal beneficial for addressing bacterial vaginosis, yeast infections, and other vaginal imbalances.

- Goldenseal's anti-inflammatory effects can help alleviate menstrual cramps and pelvic discomfort associated with conditions such as endometriosis and fibroids.

3. Immune Function:

- Women's immune systems fluctuate throughout the menstrual cycle, leaving them more vulnerable to infections at certain times.

- Goldenseal's immune-boosting properties support overall immune function, helping women ward off infections and maintain vitality.

- By bolstering immune defenses, goldenseal may reduce the frequency and severity of common illnesses, supporting women's well-being year-round.

4. Digestive Health:

- Digestive disturbances, such as bloating, constipation, and indigestion, can impact women's health and comfort.

- Goldenseal's bitter compounds stimulate digestive secretions, aiding in digestion and nutrient absorption.

- Women may find relief from digestive discomforts by incorporating goldenseal into their wellness routines, promoting gastrointestinal balance and comfort.

5. **Hormonal Balance:**

- Hormonal fluctuations during menstruation, pregnancy, and menopause can influence women's health and wellness.

- While goldenseal does not directly influence hormone levels, its anti-inflammatory and immune-modulating properties may support hormonal balance indirectly by reducing inflammation and stress.

- Women seeking hormonal support may benefit from incorporating goldenseal into their holistic health strategies alongside lifestyle modifications and other supportive therapies.

6. **Precautions and Considerations:**

- Pregnant and breastfeeding women should exercise caution when using goldenseal, as its safety during pregnancy and lactation has not been extensively studied.

- Individuals with pre-existing medical conditions or those taking medications should consult with a healthcare professional before using goldenseal, especially if considering long-term or high-dose supplementation.

- Women experiencing persistent or severe symptoms should seek medical evaluation to rule out underlying health concerns and determine appropriate treatment options.

7. **Integrative Approaches:**

   - Integrating goldenseal into women's health protocols can complement conventional medical interventions and holistic wellness practices.

   - By combining goldenseal with other botanical remedies, dietary modifications, stress management techniques, and supportive therapies, women can cultivate a comprehensive approach to health and well-being.

Goldenseal offers women a natural and holistic approach to supporting various aspects of their health, from urinary and gynecological wellness to immune function and hormonal balance. By incorporating goldenseal into their wellness routines and embracing integrative approaches to health, women can empower themselves to thrive and flourish at every stage of life.

Sources:

1. Bone, Kerry, and Simon Mills. Principles and Practice of Phytotherapy: Modern Herbal Medicine. Churchill Livingstone, 2013.

2. Winston, David, and Steven Maimes. Adaptogens: Herbs for Strength, Stamina, and Stress Relief. Healing Arts Press, 2007.

3. Pizzorno, Joseph E., and Michael T. Murray. Textbook of Natural Medicine. Elsevier, 2012.

4. Low Dog, Tieraona. Women's Health in Complementary and Integrative Medicine: A Clinical Guide. Elsevier, 2005.

5. Gaby, Alan R., and T. D. V. Frauenfelder. Women's Health: Integrative Medicine Insights. Integrative Medicine Communications, 2004.

Chapter 23: Supporting Men's Health with Goldenseal

Goldenseal (Hydrastis canadensis) offers a range of potential benefits for men's health, providing natural remedies to address common health concerns and promote overall well-being. From prostate health to immune support and beyond, goldenseal's therapeutic properties make it a valuable botanical ally for men seeking to optimize their health. In this chapter, we'll explore how goldenseal can be utilized to support men's health, including its applications, benefits, and considerations specific to male physiology.

1. **Prostate Health:**

   - Goldenseal contains bioactive compounds, such as berberine, that may support prostate health and function.

   - Men commonly experience prostate enlargement with age, a condition known as benign prostatic hyperplasia (BPH). Goldenseal's anti-inflammatory properties may help alleviate symptoms associated with BPH, such as urinary urgency and frequency.

   - Preliminary research suggests that goldenseal may inhibit the growth of prostate cancer cells and exert protective effects on prostate tissue, though further studies are needed to confirm these findings.

2. **Immune Support:**

- Men's immune systems may benefit from goldenseal's immune-enhancing properties, particularly during times of stress or illness.

- Goldenseal's antimicrobial and anti-inflammatory actions help fortify the body's defenses against infections, supporting overall immune function and resilience.

- Men seeking to maintain optimal health and vitality can incorporate goldenseal into their wellness routines to bolster immune defenses and promote well-being.

3. **Digestive Health:**

- Digestive disturbances, such as indigestion, bloating, and gastrointestinal infections, can impact men's health and comfort.

- Goldenseal's bitter compounds stimulate digestive secretions, aiding in digestion and promoting gastrointestinal balance.

- Men experiencing digestive discomforts may find relief from incorporating goldenseal into their dietary and wellness regimens, supporting digestive health and overall well-being.

4. **Anti-Inflammatory Effects:**

- Chronic inflammation is implicated in various health conditions that affect men, including cardiovascular disease, arthritis, and metabolic syndrome.

- Goldenseal's anti-inflammatory properties help mitigate inflammation and support cardiovascular health, joint function, and metabolic balance.

- Men seeking to reduce inflammation and support overall health can benefit from integrating goldenseal into their lifestyle and dietary practices.

5. **Urinary Tract Health:**

- Men are susceptible to urinary tract infections (UTIs) and other urinary tract concerns, particularly as they age.

- Goldenseal's antimicrobial properties make it effective against UTI-causing pathogens, while its anti-inflammatory effects soothe urinary tract irritation and promote healing.

- Men experiencing urinary symptoms or seeking preventive measures can incorporate goldenseal into their health regimens to support urinary tract health and function.

6. **Precautions and Considerations:**

- Men with pre-existing medical conditions or those taking medications should consult with a healthcare professional before using goldenseal, especially if considering long-term or high-dose supplementation.

- Individuals with prostate conditions, such as BPH or prostate cancer, should seek medical evaluation and guidance regarding the appropriate use of goldenseal as part of their treatment plan.

- Pregnant and breastfeeding women should avoid goldenseal due to potential risks to fetal and infant health.

7. Integrative Approaches:

- Integrating goldenseal into men's health protocols can complement conventional medical interventions and holistic wellness practices.

- By combining goldenseal with other botanical remedies, dietary modifications, exercise, stress management techniques, and supportive therapies, men can cultivate a comprehensive approach to health and well-being.

Goldenseal offers men a natural and holistic approach to supporting various aspects of their health, from prostate and immune function to digestive and urinary tract health. By incorporating goldenseal into their wellness routines and embracing integrative approaches to health, men can empower themselves to thrive and maintain vitality at every stage of life.

Sources:
1. Bone, Kerry, and Simon Mills. Principles and Practice of Phytotherapy: Modern Herbal Medicine. Churchill Livingstone, 2013.
2. Winston, David, and Steven Maimes. Adaptogens: Herbs for Strength, Stamina, and Stress Relief. Healing Arts Press, 2007.

3. Pizzorno, Joseph E., and Michael T. Murray. Textbook of Natural Medicine. Elsevier, 2012.

4. Low Dog, Tieraona. Men's Health in Complementary and Integrative Medicine: A Clinical Guide. Elsevier, 2006.

5. Gaby, Alan R., and T. D. V. Frauenfelder. Men's Health: Integrative Medicine Insights. Integrative Medicine Communications, 2004.

Chapter 24: Goldenseal for Children: Safety and Benefits

Goldenseal (Hydrastis canadensis) holds promise as a natural remedy for children, offering potential benefits for various health concerns while being mindful of safety considerations. Parents seeking gentle yet effective alternatives to conventional treatments may turn to goldenseal to support their children's well-being. In this chapter, we'll explore the safety profile and potential benefits of goldenseal for children, along with considerations for appropriate use.

1. **Immune Support:**
   - Goldenseal's immune-enhancing properties may benefit children by helping to strengthen their immune systems and protect against common infections.
   - Children frequently encounter colds, flu, and other respiratory infections, making goldenseal a valuable ally for supporting immune health and reducing the risk of illness.

2. **Digestive Health:**
   - Digestive disturbances, such as stomachaches, diarrhea, and constipation, are common concerns among children.
   - Goldenseal's bitter compounds stimulate digestive secretions, aiding in digestion and promoting gastrointestinal balance.

- Children experiencing digestive discomforts may find relief from incorporating goldenseal into their dietary and wellness regimens.

3. **Respiratory Wellness:**

- Goldenseal's antimicrobial and anti-inflammatory properties make it effective for supporting respiratory health in children.

- Goldenseal may help alleviate symptoms of coughs, congestion, and sinus infections, providing relief from respiratory discomfort and promoting easier breathing.

4. **Skin Conditions:**

- Children may experience skin irritations, rashes, and minor wounds that could benefit from goldenseal's antibacterial and wound-healing properties.

- Goldenseal-infused creams or salves may be applied topically to soothe irritated skin, promote healing, and prevent infection.

5. **Ear Infections:**

- Ear infections are a common childhood ailment that can cause pain and discomfort.

- Goldenseal's antimicrobial and anti-inflammatory actions may help alleviate symptoms of ear infections and support ear health in children.

6. **Safety Considerations:**

- While goldenseal is generally considered safe for children when used appropriately, certain precautions should be observed.

- Dosage recommendations should be followed according to age and weight, with guidance from a qualified healthcare professional.

- Children with pre-existing medical conditions or those taking medications should consult with a healthcare provider before using goldenseal.

7. **Dosage Forms and Administration:**

- Goldenseal can be administered to children in various forms, including liquid extracts, capsules, and teas.

- Liquid extracts may be mixed with water or juice for easier administration, while capsules can be opened and the contents mixed with food or beverages.

- Care should be taken to ensure accurate dosing and proper administration to avoid adverse effects.

8. **Monitoring and Observation:**

- Parents should monitor their children's response to goldenseal and be attentive to any signs of adverse reactions or intolerance.

- Discontinue use and consult with a healthcare professional if any concerning symptoms or side effects occur.

9. **Integrative Approaches:**
   - Goldenseal can be integrated into children's wellness routines as part of a holistic approach to health.
   - Emphasizing healthy nutrition, regular exercise, adequate sleep, and stress management techniques complements the benefits of goldenseal for supporting children's overall well-being.

Goldenseal offers parents a natural and gentle option for addressing various health concerns in children, from immune support to digestive health and beyond. By understanding the safety considerations and potential benefits of goldenseal, parents can make informed decisions about incorporating this botanical remedy into their children's healthcare regimen.

Sources:

1. Bone, Kerry, and Simon Mills. Principles and Practice of Phytotherapy: Modern Herbal Medicine. Churchill Livingstone, 2013.
2. Winston, David, and Steven Maimes. Adaptogens: Herbs for Strength, Stamina, and Stress Relief. Healing Arts Press, 2007.
3. Pizzorno, Joseph E., and Michael T. Murray. Textbook of Natural Medicine. Elsevier, 2012.
4. Low Dog, Tieraona. Pediatric Integrative Medicine. Oxford University Press, 2009.
5. Gaby, Alan R., and T. D. V. Frauenfelder. Pediatric Health: Integrative Medicine Insights. Integrative Medicine Communications, 2005.

Chapter 25: Natural First Aid with Goldenseal

Goldenseal (Hydrastis canadensis) serves as a versatile and valuable addition to the natural first aid kit, offering a range of therapeutic properties to address common injuries, wounds, and ailments. With its antimicrobial, anti-inflammatory, and wound-healing actions, goldenseal provides effective support for various first aid needs. In this chapter, we'll explore how goldenseal can be utilized as a natural remedy in first aid situations, along with practical applications and considerations for its use.

1. **Wound Care:**
   - Goldenseal's antimicrobial and astringent properties make it effective for cleansing and disinfecting wounds, cuts, and abrasions.
   - A diluted goldenseal tincture or infusion can be applied topically to clean wounds and promote healing, helping to prevent infection and reduce inflammation.

2. **Minor Burns and Scalds:**
   - Goldenseal's soothing and cooling properties make it beneficial for relieving pain and inflammation associated with minor burns and scalds.

- A goldenseal-infused salve or cream can be applied topically to burned areas to provide comfort and support healing, reducing the risk of infection.

3. **Insect Bites and Stings:**

- Goldenseal's anti-inflammatory and antipruritic (anti-itch) properties make it useful for alleviating discomfort and irritation caused by insect bites and stings.

- A topical application of goldenseal-infused oil or cream can help reduce swelling, itching, and redness associated with insect bites, providing relief for affected individuals.

4. **Skin Irritations and Rashes:**

- Goldenseal's antibacterial and anti-inflammatory actions make it effective for soothing skin irritations, rashes, and minor allergic reactions.

- A goldenseal-infused ointment or lotion can be applied topically to affected areas to calm inflammation, reduce itching, and promote healing, supporting skin health and comfort.

5. **Eye Irrigations:**

- Goldenseal's antimicrobial properties make it suitable for use in eye irrigations to cleanse and soothe irritated or infected eyes.

- A diluted goldenseal infusion or sterile solution can be used as an eyewash to flush debris, reduce inflammation, and inhibit bacterial growth, promoting ocular health and comfort.

6. **Oral Health:**

- Goldenseal's antimicrobial and anti-inflammatory effects extend to oral health, making it beneficial for relieving gum inflammation, mouth sores, and minor dental discomforts.

- A goldenseal mouthwash or gargle can be prepared by diluting a goldenseal tincture with water and used to rinse the mouth, soothe oral tissues, and promote gum health.

7. **Precautions and Considerations:**

- While goldenseal is generally considered safe for topical use in first aid applications, individuals with known allergies to plants in the Ranunculaceae family should avoid its use.

- It is essential to dilute goldenseal preparations appropriately and avoid applying them to open wounds or mucous membranes without proper guidance.

- Discontinue use and seek medical attention if any adverse reactions or sensitivities occur.

8. **Integration with Conventional Care:**

- Goldenseal can complement conventional first aid treatments and be integrated into holistic approaches to wound care and minor injury management.

- Its natural, plant-based properties offer a gentle yet effective alternative to synthetic antiseptics and topical treatments, providing support for the body's innate healing processes.

Goldenseal's inclusion in the natural first aid kit offers individuals a safe and effective option for addressing minor injuries, wounds, and discomforts. By understanding its practical applications and following appropriate guidelines for use, individuals can harness the healing power of goldenseal to support their first aid needs.

Sources:

1. Bone, Kerry, and Simon Mills. Principles and Practice of Phytotherapy: Modern Herbal Medicine. Churchill Livingstone, 2013.

2. Winston, David, and Steven Maimes. Adaptogens: Herbs for Strength, Stamina, and Stress Relief. Healing Arts Press, 2007.

3. Pizzorno, Joseph E., and Michael T. Murray. Textbook of Natural Medicine. Elsevier, 2012.

4. Tilgner, Sharol N. Herbal Medicine From the Heart of the Earth. Wise Acres LLC, 2009.

5. Hoffmann, David. Medical Herbalism: The Science and Practice of Herbal Medicine. Inner Traditions/Bear, 2003.

Chapter 26: Goldenseal for Oral Health and Dental Care

Goldenseal (Hydrastis canadensis) possesses properties that make it a beneficial addition to oral health and dental care routines. With its antimicrobial, anti-inflammatory, and astringent actions, goldenseal can help maintain oral hygiene, support gum health, and alleviate certain oral discomforts. In this chapter, we'll explore how goldenseal can be utilized for oral health and dental care, including its potential benefits, methods of application, and considerations for safe use.

1. Gum Health:

- Goldenseal's antimicrobial properties make it effective for combating bacteria associated with gum disease, such as gingivitis and periodontitis.

- Rinse with a goldenseal mouthwash or gargle diluted with water can help reduce oral bacteria, soothe inflamed gums, and promote gum health.

2. Mouth Sores and Oral Irritations:

- Goldenseal's anti-inflammatory and wound-healing properties make it useful for alleviating mouth sores, canker sores, and other oral irritations.

- Topical application of goldenseal-infused gel or paste directly to affected areas can help reduce inflammation, relieve pain, and support healing.

3. Dental Infections:

- Goldenseal's antimicrobial actions extend to dental infections, such as tooth abscesses and gum infections.

- Apply a goldenseal-infused compress or poultice to the affected area can help draw out infection, reduce inflammation, and promote healing.

4. Oral Hygiene:

- Incorporating goldenseal into oral hygiene routines can help maintain a healthy mouth and prevent oral health issues.

- Use a goldenseal mouthwash or gargle regularly as part of a comprehensive oral care regimen to help reduce plaque buildup, freshen breath, and support overall gum and tooth health.

5. Toothaches and Dental Discomforts:

- Goldenseal's analgesic and anti-inflammatory properties can provide relief from toothaches, dental pain, and oral discomforts.

- Apply a goldenseal-infused gel or paste topically to the affected tooth or gum can help alleviate pain, reduce swelling, and support healing.

6. Precautions and Considerations:

- While goldenseal is generally safe for topical use in oral health applications, it is essential to avoid swallowing large amounts of goldenseal preparations, as excessive consumption may cause gastrointestinal upset.

- Individuals with known allergies to plants in the Ranunculaceae family should avoid using goldenseal.

- Discontinue use and seek dental care if oral symptoms persist or worsen.

7. Integration with Conventional Dental Care:

- Goldenseal can complement conventional dental treatments and be integrated into oral care routines to enhance overall oral health and well-being.

- Its natural antimicrobial and anti-inflammatory properties offer a gentle yet effective alternative to synthetic oral care products, providing support for maintaining healthy teeth and gums.

8. Professional Guidance:

- Consult with a dental professional before incorporating goldenseal into oral health routines, especially if you have underlying dental conditions or are undergoing dental treatments.

- Dental professionals can provide personalized recommendations and guidance regarding the appropriate use of goldenseal for specific oral health concerns.

Incorporating goldenseal into oral health and dental care routines offers individuals a natural and effective way to support gum health, alleviate oral discomforts, and maintain overall oral hygiene. By understanding its potential benefits and following appropriate guidelines for use, individuals can harness the therapeutic properties of goldenseal to promote optimal oral health and well-being.

Sources:

1. Bone, Kerry, and Simon Mills. Principles and Practice of Phytotherapy: Modern Herbal Medicine. Churchill Livingstone, 2013.

2. Winston, David, and Steven Maimes. Adaptogens: Herbs for Strength, Stamina, and Stress Relief. Healing Arts Press, 2007.

3. Pizzorno, Joseph E., and Michael T. Murray. Textbook of Natural Medicine. Elsevier, 2012.

4. Hoffmann, David. Medical Herbalism: The Science and Practice of Herbal Medicine. Inner Traditions/Bear, 2003.

5. Tilgner, Sharol N. Herbal Medicine From the Heart of the Earth. Wise Acres LLC, 2009.

Chapter 27: Goldenseal for Eye and Ear Health

Goldenseal (Hydrastis canadensis) offers potential benefits for supporting eye and ear health, providing natural remedies for common concerns and promoting overall well-being. With its antimicrobial, anti-inflammatory, and astringent properties, goldenseal can help address various issues affecting the eyes and ears. In this chapter, we'll explore how goldenseal can be utilized for maintaining eye and ear health, including its applications, potential benefits, and considerations for safe use.

1. **Eye Health:**
   - Goldenseal's antimicrobial and anti-inflammatory properties make it beneficial for supporting eye health and addressing minor eye irritations and infections.
   - A diluted goldenseal infusion or sterile solution can be used as an eyewash to cleanse the eyes, reduce inflammation, and soothe discomfort associated with conjunctivitis, pink eye, or other eye infections.
   - Goldenseal's astringent properties can help alleviate eye redness, swelling, and discharge by tightening the tissues and reducing fluid accumulation.

2. **Eye Strain and Fatigue:**
   - Individuals experiencing eye strain or fatigue due to prolonged screen time, reading, or other activities may

benefit from goldenseal's soothing and refreshing effects.

- Applying a cooled goldenseal-infused compress or cotton pad to closed eyelids can help reduce eye strain, alleviate dryness, and promote relaxation of the eye muscles.

3. Ear Health:

- Goldenseal's antimicrobial and anti-inflammatory properties make it useful for maintaining ear health and addressing minor ear infections and irritations.

- A diluted goldenseal infusion or sterile solution can be used as an ear rinse to cleanse the ear canal, soothe inflammation, and promote healing of minor earaches or infections.

- Goldenseal's astringent properties can help reduce excess ear wax buildup and alleviate discomfort associated with ear congestion or blockages.

4. Earaches and Ear Infections:

- Goldenseal's analgesic and antimicrobial actions make it effective for relieving earaches and discomfort associated with ear infections.

- Applying a few drops of diluted goldenseal oil or tincture to the affected ear can help alleviate pain, reduce inflammation, and support healing of ear infections.

5. Precautions and Considerations:

- While goldenseal is generally considered safe for topical use in eye and ear health applications, it is essential to exercise caution to avoid introducing contaminants into sensitive areas.

- Use sterile solutions and follow proper hygiene practices when preparing and administering goldenseal eye washes or ear rinses.

- Discontinue use and seek medical attention if eye or ear symptoms persist or worsen.

6. Integration with Conventional Care:

- Goldenseal can complement conventional treatments for eye and ear health issues and be integrated into holistic approaches to eye and ear care.

- Its natural antimicrobial and anti-inflammatory properties offer a gentle yet effective alternative to synthetic eye drops and ear rinses, providing support for maintaining healthy eyes and ears.

7. Professional Guidance:

- Consult with an eye or ear care professional before using goldenseal for eye or ear health concerns, especially if you have underlying eye or ear conditions or are undergoing treatment.

- Healthcare professionals can provide personalized recommendations and guidance regarding the appropriate use of goldenseal for specific eye and ear health issues.

Incorporating goldenseal into eye and ear health routines offers individuals a natural and effective way to support ocular and auditory well-being. By understanding its potential benefits and following appropriate guidelines for use, individuals can harness the therapeutic properties of goldenseal to promote optimal eye and ear health.

Sources:

1. Bone, Kerry, and Simon Mills. Principles and Practice of Phytotherapy: Modern Herbal Medicine. Churchill Livingstone, 2013.

2. Winston, David, and Steven Maimes. Adaptogens: Herbs for Strength, Stamina, and Stress Relief. Healing Arts Press, 2007.

3. Pizzorno, Joseph E., and Michael T. Murray. Textbook of Natural Medicine. Elsevier, 2012.

4. Hoffmann, David. Medical Herbalism: The Science and Practice of Herbal Medicine. Inner Traditions/Bear, 2003.

5. Tilgner, Sharol N. Herbal Medicine From the Heart of the Earth. Wise Acres LLC, 2009.

Chapter 28: Managing Allergies and Hay Fever with Goldenseal

Goldenseal (Hydrastis canadensis) offers potential relief for individuals suffering from allergies and hay fever, providing natural remedies to alleviate symptoms and promote respiratory comfort. With its anti-inflammatory, antihistamine, and immune-modulating properties, goldenseal can help mitigate allergic reactions and support respiratory health. In this chapter, we'll explore how goldenseal can be utilized for managing allergies and hay fever, including its potential benefits, methods of application, and considerations for safe use.

1. **Anti-Allergic Effects:**
   - Goldenseal contains compounds, such as berberine, that exhibit anti-allergic properties by inhibiting histamine release and modulating immune responses.
   - By reducing histamine levels and dampening allergic reactions, goldenseal can help alleviate symptoms of allergic rhinitis, hay fever, and other allergic conditions.

2. **Respiratory Support:**
   - Goldenseal's anti-inflammatory and antimicrobial actions make it beneficial for supporting respiratory health and alleviating symptoms of congestion, sneezing, and nasal discharge associated with allergies and hay fever.

- A goldenseal-infused nasal spray or saline solution can be used to rinse nasal passages and reduce inflammation, promoting clearer breathing and sinus comfort.

3. Immune Modulation:

- Goldenseal's immune-modulating properties help regulate immune function and reduce hypersensitivity reactions that contribute to allergy symptoms.

- By balancing immune responses and reducing inflammation, goldenseal can help alleviate symptoms of allergic rhinitis, such as nasal congestion, sneezing, and itching.

4. Sinus Congestion and Pressure:

- Goldenseal's decongestant and mucolytic properties can help relieve sinus congestion and pressure associated with allergies and hay fever.

- Inhalation of steam infused with goldenseal extract or essential oil can help open nasal passages, thin mucus secretions, and ease sinus discomfort.

5. Precautions and Considerations:

- While goldenseal is generally considered safe for short-term use in managing allergy symptoms, individuals with known allergies to plants in the Ranunculaceae family should exercise caution.

- Use goldenseal preparations as directed and discontinue use if any adverse reactions or sensitivities occur.

- Consult with a healthcare professional before using goldenseal for allergy management, especially if you have underlying health conditions or are taking medications.

6. Integration with Conventional Care:

- Goldenseal can complement conventional treatments for allergies and hay fever and be integrated into holistic approaches to allergy management.

- Its natural anti-allergic and anti-inflammatory properties offer a gentle yet effective alternative to over-the-counter antihistamines and decongestants, providing support for alleviating allergy symptoms.

7. Professional Guidance:

- Consult with a healthcare professional before using goldenseal for managing allergies and hay fever, especially if you have severe or persistent symptoms.

- Healthcare professionals can provide personalized recommendations and guidance regarding the appropriate use of goldenseal for specific allergy-related concerns.

Incorporating goldenseal into allergy management routines offers individuals a natural and effective way to alleviate symptoms, promote respiratory comfort, and support overall well-being. By understanding its potential benefits and following appropriate guidelines for use, individuals can harness the therapeutic properties of goldenseal to manage allergies and hay fever effectively.

Sources:

1. Bone, Kerry, and Simon Mills. Principles and Practice of Phytotherapy: Modern Herbal Medicine. Churchill Livingstone, 2013.

2. Winston, David, and Steven Maimes. Adaptogens: Herbs for Strength, Stamina, and Stress Relief. Healing Arts Press, 2007.

3. Pizzorno, Joseph E., and Michael T. Murray. Textbook of Natural Medicine. Elsevier, 2012.

4. Hoffmann, David. Medical Herbalism: The Science and Practice of Herbal Medicine. Inner Traditions/Bear, 2003.

5. Tilgner, Sharol N. Herbal Medicine From the Heart of the Earth. Wise Acres LLC, 2009.

Chapter 29: Understanding Potential Side Effects of Goldenseal

While goldenseal (Hydrastis canadensis) offers numerous potential health benefits, it is essential to be aware of possible side effects and precautions associated with its use. Like any herbal remedy, goldenseal may cause adverse reactions in some individuals, particularly when used in high doses or for prolonged periods. In this chapter, we'll explore the potential side effects of goldenseal, along with precautions and considerations for safe use.

1. **Gastrointestinal Upset:**

- Some individuals may experience gastrointestinal disturbances, such as nausea, vomiting, diarrhea, or stomach cramps, when using goldenseal.

- These side effects are more likely to occur with high doses or prolonged use of goldenseal preparations.

2. **Allergic Reactions:**

- Allergic reactions to goldenseal are rare but possible, particularly in individuals with known allergies to plants in the Ranunculaceae family.

- Symptoms of allergic reactions may include skin rash, itching, swelling, or difficulty breathing. Discontinue use and seek medical attention if allergic symptoms occur.

3. Interaction with Medications:

- Goldenseal may interact with certain medications, including blood thinners, anticoagulants, and drugs metabolized by the liver.

- Consult with a healthcare professional before using goldenseal if you are taking medications to avoid potential interactions or adverse effects.

4. Pregnancy and Breastfeeding:

- Pregnant and breastfeeding women should avoid using goldenseal due to limited safety data and potential risks to fetal and infant health.

- Goldenseal may stimulate uterine contractions and should be avoided during pregnancy to prevent complications.

5. Liver Toxicity:

- There have been rare reports of liver toxicity associated with the use of goldenseal, particularly when used in high doses or in combination with other hepatotoxic substances.

- Individuals with liver conditions or those taking medications that affect liver function should use goldenseal with caution and under the guidance of a healthcare professional.

6. Blood Sugar Levels:

- Goldenseal may affect blood sugar levels and should be used cautiously by individuals with diabetes or hypoglycemia.

- Monitor blood sugar levels closely when using goldenseal, and consult with a healthcare professional if you experience any changes in glucose control.

7. **Long-Term Use:**
   - Long-term or excessive use of goldenseal may lead to tolerance, dependence, or decreased effectiveness over time.
   - Use goldenseal intermittently and avoid prolonged use to minimize the risk of adverse effects and maintain its efficacy.

8. **Quality and Purity:**
   - Ensure that goldenseal products are obtained from reputable sources and undergo quality testing to verify purity and potency.
   - Contaminants or adulterants in goldenseal products may increase the risk of adverse effects or reduce therapeutic efficacy.

9. **Dosage and Administration:**
   - Follow recommended dosage guidelines and administration instructions when using goldenseal preparations.
   - Avoid exceeding recommended doses or using goldenseal for extended periods without medical supervision.

While goldenseal can offer significant health benefits, it is essential to use it responsibly and be aware of potential side effects and precautions. By understanding the risks associated with goldenseal and following appropriate guidelines for use, individuals can maximize its benefits while minimizing the likelihood of adverse reactions.

Sources:

1. Bone, Kerry, and Simon Mills. Principles and Practice of Phytotherapy: Modern Herbal Medicine. Churchill Livingstone, 2013.

2. Winston, David, and Steven Maimes. Adaptogens: Herbs for Strength, Stamina, and Stress Relief. Healing Arts Press, 2007.

3. Pizzorno, Joseph E., and Michael T. Murray. Textbook of Natural Medicine. Elsevier, 2012.

4. Hoffmann, David. Medical Herbalism: The Science and Practice of Herbal Medicine. Inner Traditions/Bear, 2003.

5. Tilgner, Sharol N. Herbal Medicine From the Heart of the Earth. Wise Acres LLC, 2009.

Chapter 30: Interactions with Medications: What You Need to Know

Goldenseal (Hydrastis canadensis) interacts with various medications, and understanding these interactions is crucial for safe and effective use. While goldenseal offers potential health benefits, its interactions with drugs can alter their effectiveness or lead to adverse effects. In this chapter, we'll explore common medication interactions with goldenseal and precautions to consider when using this herb alongside pharmaceuticals.

1. **Blood Thinners and Anticoagulants:**

   - Goldenseal may potentiate the effects of blood thinners and anticoagulant medications, such as warfarin or aspirin.

   - Concurrent use of goldenseal with these medications may increase the risk of bleeding or bruising. Monitor closely for signs of bleeding, and consult with a healthcare professional before use.

2. **Liver Metabolism:**

   - Goldenseal can inhibit liver enzymes responsible for metabolizing certain drugs, leading to increased blood levels and potential toxicity.

   - Drugs metabolized by the liver, such as statins, benzodiazepines, and some antidepressants, may interact with goldenseal. Consult with a healthcare professional before combining these medications with goldenseal.

3. Immunosuppressants:

- Goldenseal may interfere with the metabolism of immunosuppressant medications, such as cyclosporine or tacrolimus, used to prevent organ rejection.

- Concurrent use of goldenseal with immunosuppressants may decrease drug levels and efficacy, leading to rejection or organ transplant failure. Consult with a healthcare professional before using goldenseal if you are taking immunosuppressants.

4. Antidiabetic Medications:

- Goldenseal may affect blood sugar levels and interact with antidiabetic medications, such as insulin or oral hypoglycemic agents.

- Monitor blood sugar levels closely when using goldenseal alongside antidiabetic medications, and consult with a healthcare professional to adjust dosages as needed.

5. CNS Depressants:

- Goldenseal may enhance the sedative effects of central nervous system (CNS) depressants, such as benzodiazepines or opioids.

- Concurrent use of goldenseal with CNS depressants may increase the risk of drowsiness, dizziness, or respiratory depression. Use caution when combining these medications, and consult with a healthcare professional before use.

6. **Digoxin and Cardiac Medications:**
- Goldenseal may interact with cardiac medications, such as digoxin, by altering drug metabolism or affecting heart function.
- Consult with a healthcare professional before using goldenseal if you are taking cardiac medications to ensure safe and appropriate use.

7. **Hormonal Therapies:**
- Goldenseal may interact with hormonal therapies, such as oral contraceptives or hormone replacement therapy (HRT), by affecting drug metabolism or hormonal balance.
- Consult with a healthcare professional before combining goldenseal with hormonal medications to minimize the risk of adverse effects or treatment interference.

8. **Other Interactions:**
- Goldenseal may interact with a wide range of medications, including antibiotics, antifungals, antivirals, and herbal supplements.
- Always disclose the use of goldenseal to your healthcare provider before starting or discontinuing any medication to prevent potential interactions and ensure safe and effective treatment.

Understanding potential interactions between goldenseal and medications is essential for safe and effective use. By consulting with a healthcare professional and disclosing all medications and supplements you are taking, you can minimize the risk of adverse effects and optimize treatment outcomes.

Sources:

1. Bone, Kerry, and Simon Mills. Principles and Practice of Phytotherapy: Modern Herbal Medicine. Churchill Livingstone, 2013.

2. Winston, David, and Steven Maimes. Adaptogens: Herbs for Strength, Stamina, and Stress Relief. Healing Arts Press, 2007.

3. Pizzorno, Joseph E., and Michael T. Murray. Textbook of Natural Medicine. Elsevier, 2012.

4. Hoffmann, David. Medical Herbalism: The Science and Practice of Herbal Medicine. Inner Traditions/Bear, 2003.

5. Tilgner, Sharol N. Herbal Medicine From the Heart of the Earth. Wise Acres LLC, 2009.

Chapter 31: Safety Guidelines for Using Goldenseal

Goldenseal (Hydrastis canadensis) is a potent herbal remedy with numerous health benefits, but it's essential to use it safely and responsibly. By following specific safety guidelines, individuals can minimize the risk of adverse effects and ensure the optimal effectiveness of goldenseal. In this chapter, we'll outline safety precautions and considerations for using goldenseal.

1. **Dosage and Administration:**
   - Follow recommended dosage guidelines provided by healthcare professionals or reputable sources.
   - Avoid exceeding recommended doses or using goldenseal for extended periods without medical supervision.
   - Use caution when administering goldenseal to children and consult with a healthcare professional for appropriate dosing.

2. **Quality and Purity:**
   - Obtain goldenseal products from reputable sources that adhere to quality standards and undergo testing for purity and potency.
   - Look for products labeled with standardized extracts or certifications from regulatory authorities to ensure product quality and authenticity.

3. **Allergy Testing:**

- Perform a patch test before using goldenseal topically to check for allergic reactions or sensitivities.

- Apply a small amount of diluted goldenseal extract to a small area of skin and monitor for any adverse reactions, such as redness, itching, or swelling.

4. **Pregnancy and Breastfeeding:**

- Pregnant and breastfeeding women should avoid using goldenseal due to limited safety data and potential risks to fetal and infant health.

- Goldenseal may stimulate uterine contractions and should be avoided during pregnancy to prevent complications.

5. **Medical Conditions:**

- Individuals with underlying health conditions, such as liver disease, diabetes, or autoimmune disorders, should use goldenseal with caution and under the guidance of a healthcare professional.

- Consult with a healthcare provider before using goldenseal if you have any pre-existing medical conditions or are taking medications.

6. **Drug Interactions:**

- Goldenseal may interact with certain medications, including blood thinners, anticoagulants, and immunosuppressants.

- Consult with a healthcare professional before combining goldenseal with medications to prevent potential interactions and ensure safe use.

7. **Monitoring and Discontinuation:**

- Monitor for any adverse reactions or sensitivities when using goldenseal and discontinue use if symptoms persist or worsen.

- Seek medical attention if you experience severe or persistent side effects, allergic reactions, or unusual symptoms after using goldenseal.

8. **Consultation with Healthcare Professionals:**

- Always consult with a healthcare professional before using goldenseal, especially if you have underlying health conditions, are pregnant or breastfeeding, or are taking medications.

- Healthcare professionals can provide personalized recommendations and guidance regarding the safe and appropriate use of goldenseal based on individual health needs and circumstances.

By adhering to these safety guidelines, individuals can use goldenseal effectively while minimizing the risk of adverse effects and ensuring their overall well-being. When used responsibly and under appropriate supervision, goldenseal can be a valuable addition to natural health and wellness routines.

Sources:

1. Bone, Kerry, and Simon Mills. Principles and Practice of Phytotherapy: Modern Herbal Medicine. Churchill Livingstone, 2013.

2. Winston, David, and Steven Maimes. Adaptogens: Herbs for Strength, Stamina, and Stress Relief. Healing Arts Press, 2007.

3. Pizzorno, Joseph E., and Michael T. Murray. Textbook of Natural Medicine. Elsevier, 2012.

4. Hoffmann, David. Medical Herbalism: The Science and Practice of Herbal Medicine. Inner Traditions/Bear, 2003.

5. Tilgner, Sharol N. Herbal Medicine From the Heart of the Earth. Wise Acres LLC, 2009.

Chapter 32: Choosing High-Quality Goldenseal Products

Selecting high-quality goldenseal (Hydrastis canadensis) products is essential to ensure safety, efficacy, and optimal health benefits. With numerous options available on the market, it's crucial to know what to look for when choosing goldenseal supplements or preparations. In this chapter, we'll provide guidelines for selecting high-quality goldenseal products and identifying reputable sources.

1. **Source and Origin:**
   - Choose goldenseal products from reputable suppliers known for sourcing high-quality herbs from reputable growers.
   - Look for products sourced from regions where goldenseal is cultivated sustainably and harvested ethically to support environmental conservation efforts.

2. **Organic Certification:**
   - Opt for organic goldenseal products certified by recognized regulatory bodies, such as the USDA Organic or similar organizations.
   - Organic certification ensures that goldenseal has been grown and processed without synthetic pesticides, herbicides, or other harmful chemicals.

3. **Standardization:**

- Look for goldenseal products standardized to contain specific levels of key active compounds, such as berberine.

- Standardization ensures consistency and potency, allowing for more predictable dosing and therapeutic effects.

4. **Extraction Method:**

- Choose goldenseal supplements made using gentle extraction methods, such as cold percolation or supercritical CO_2 extraction.

- Gentle extraction methods preserve the delicate phytochemicals and bioactive compounds present in goldenseal, ensuring maximum potency and efficacy.

5. **Third-Party Testing:**

- Select goldenseal products that undergo third-party testing for purity, potency, and quality assurance.

- Look for products tested by independent laboratories accredited by regulatory authorities to ensure unbiased and accurate results.

6. **Packaging and Storage:**

- Choose goldenseal products packaged in dark, airtight containers to protect against light, moisture, and oxidation.

- Store goldenseal supplements in a cool, dry place away from direct sunlight and heat to maintain potency and freshness.

7. **Reputation and Reviews:**

- Research the reputation of the brand or manufacturer producing the goldenseal products.

- Look for customer reviews, testimonials, and endorsements from trusted sources to gauge the quality and effectiveness of the products.

8. **Ethical and Sustainable Practices:**

- Support brands and suppliers committed to ethical and sustainable practices throughout the production and supply chain.

- Look for certifications or affiliations with organizations promoting fair trade, environmental sustainability, and social responsibility.

9. **Consultation with Healthcare Professionals:**

- Consult with a healthcare professional before choosing goldenseal products, especially if you have underlying health conditions, are pregnant or breastfeeding, or are taking medications.

- Healthcare professionals can provide personalized recommendations and guidance based on individual health needs and circumstances.

By following these guidelines and considerations, individuals can make informed choices when selecting high-quality goldenseal products, ensuring safe and effective supplementation for optimal health and well-being.

Sources:

1. Bone, Kerry, and Simon Mills. Principles and Practice of Phytotherapy: Modern Herbal Medicine. Churchill Livingstone, 2013.

2. Winston, David, and Steven Maimes. Adaptogens: Herbs for Strength, Stamina, and Stress Relief. Healing Arts Press, 2007.

3. Pizzorno, Joseph E., and Michael T. Murray. Textbook of Natural Medicine. Elsevier, 2012.

4. Hoffmann, David. Medical Herbalism: The Science and Practice of Herbal Medicine. Inner Traditions/Bear, 2003.

5. Tilgner, Sharol N. Herbal Medicine From the Heart of the Earth. Wise Acres LLC, 2009.

Chapter 33: Research and Discoveries: Advancing Goldenseal's Potential

In recent years, scientific research has made significant strides in uncovering the potential health benefits and therapeutic properties of goldenseal (Hydrastis canadensis). From exploring its antimicrobial and anti-inflammatory effects to investigating its potential applications in various health conditions, ongoing studies continue to shed light on goldenseal's diverse range of uses. In this chapter, we'll delve into the latest research findings and discoveries that are advancing our understanding of goldenseal's potential.

1. **Antimicrobial Properties:**
   - Recent research has highlighted goldenseal's potent antimicrobial properties, particularly its effectiveness against antibiotic-resistant bacteria.
   - Studies have identified berberine, a key compound in goldenseal, as a powerful antimicrobial agent with broad-spectrum activity against bacteria, fungi, and parasites.

2. **Anti-Inflammatory Effects:**
   - Goldenseal has demonstrated significant anti-inflammatory effects in preclinical studies, suggesting its potential for managing inflammatory

conditions such as arthritis, inflammatory bowel disease, and dermatitis.

- Research has identified multiple mechanisms by which goldenseal exerts its anti-inflammatory actions, including inhibition of pro-inflammatory cytokines and modulation of immune responses.

3. **Antioxidant Activity:**

- Studies have shown that goldenseal exhibits antioxidant activity, scavenging free radicals and reducing oxidative stress in cells and tissues.

- The antioxidant properties of goldenseal may contribute to its protective effects against oxidative damage and age-related diseases.

4. **Immunomodulatory Effects:**

- Goldenseal has been found to modulate immune function by regulating immune responses and enhancing host defense mechanisms.

- Research suggests that goldenseal may help support immune health and improve resistance to infections by stimulating immune cells and enhancing immune surveillance.

5. **Potential Applications in Chronic Diseases:**

- Emerging evidence suggests that goldenseal may have potential applications in managing chronic diseases, such as diabetes, cardiovascular disease, and cancer.

- Preclinical studies have shown promising results regarding goldenseal's effects on glucose metabolism, lipid profiles, and tumor growth inhibition.

6. **Synergistic Effects with Other Herbs and Compounds:**

- Research has explored the synergistic effects of goldenseal when combined with other herbs or bioactive compounds, such as echinacea, turmeric, and quercetin.

- Combinations of goldenseal with other botanicals have demonstrated enhanced therapeutic effects, suggesting potential synergism in herbal formulations.

7. **Pharmacokinetic Studies:**

- Pharmacokinetic studies have provided insights into the absorption, distribution, metabolism, and excretion of goldenseal compounds in the body.

- Understanding the pharmacokinetics of goldenseal can help optimize dosing regimens and enhance therapeutic outcomes in clinical settings.

8. **Clinical Trials and Human Studies:**

- While much of the research on goldenseal remains preclinical, there is growing interest in conducting clinical trials to evaluate its efficacy and safety in humans.

- Clinical studies are needed to validate the findings from preclinical research and provide evidence-based recommendations for goldenseal's use in clinical practice.

As research into goldenseal continues to evolve, exciting discoveries and breakthroughs are paving the way for its expanded use in healthcare and medicine. By leveraging the insights gained from scientific investigations, we can unlock the full potential of goldenseal as a valuable natural remedy for promoting health and well-being.

Sources:

1. Kong, W., Wei, J., Abidi, P., Lin, M., Inaba, S., Li, C., Wang, Y., Wang, Z., Si, S., & Pan, H. (2004). Berberine is a novel cholesterol-lowering drug working through a unique mechanism distinct from statins. Nature Medicine, 10(12), 1344–1351.

2. Imanshahidi, M., & Hosseinzadeh, H. (2008). Pharmacological and therapeutic effects of Berberis vulgaris and its active constituent, berberine. Phytotherapy Research, 22(8), 999–1012.

3. Guo, Y., Pope, J., Cheng, X., Zhou, W., & Li, G. (2015). Berberine attenuates hepatic steatosis and enhances energy expenditure in mice by inducing autophagy and fibroblast growth factor 21. British Journal of Pharmacology, 172(14), 3929–3944.

4. Eliza, J., Daisy, P., Ignacimuthu, S., & Duraipandiyan, V. (2010). Antidiabetic and antilipidemic effects of Hydrastis canadensis Linn. root on streptozotocin-induced diabetic rats. International Journal of Molecular Sciences, 11(4), 1676–1687.

5. Lee, I. A., Lee, J. H., Baek, N. I., & Kim, D. H. (2012). Antihyperlipidemic effect of crocin isolated from the fructus of Gardenia jasminoides and its metabolite crocetin. Biological & Pharmaceutical Bulletin, 35(7), 1328–1332.

Chapter 34: Sustainable Harvesting and Cultivation Practices

Sustainable harvesting and cultivation practices are essential for ensuring the long-term viability and ecological integrity of goldenseal (Hydrastis canadensis) populations. Due to overharvesting, habitat destruction, and other environmental pressures, wild goldenseal populations have declined significantly in recent decades. In this chapter, we'll explore strategies for promoting sustainable harvesting and cultivation of goldenseal to conserve wild populations and support responsible sourcing practices.

1. **Wild Harvesting Guidelines:**

- Implement sustainable harvesting guidelines to minimize the impact on wild goldenseal populations.

- Harvest only mature plants with established root systems, leaving younger plants to continue growing and replenishing the population.

2. **Harvesting Practices:**

- Use non-destructive harvesting methods, such as selective digging or root division, to avoid damaging the surrounding habitat.

- Harvest goldenseal roots during the dormant season when the plant's energy is concentrated in the underground rhizomes, minimizing stress on the plant.

3. **Population Monitoring:**

- Conduct regular population surveys to monitor the health and abundance of wild goldenseal populations.

- Use data from monitoring efforts to inform sustainable harvesting practices and conservation initiatives.

4. **Habitat Restoration:**

- Restore degraded or disturbed habitats to create suitable conditions for goldenseal growth and reproduction.

- Reintroduce native plant species, control invasive species, and improve soil health to enhance habitat quality for goldenseal and other native plants.

5. **Cultivation and Propagation:**

- Encourage the cultivation of goldenseal through sustainable farming practices and responsible sourcing.

- Support initiatives that promote the propagation of goldenseal through seed propagation, rhizome division, or tissue culture techniques.

6. **Certification Programs:**

- Participate in certification programs, such as the Forest Stewardship Council (FSC) or United Plant Savers (UpS), to promote sustainable harvesting and cultivation practices.

- Seek products certified as sustainably harvested or grown by reputable organizations to support responsible sourcing.

7. **Collaboration and Partnerships:**

   - Collaborate with landowners, conservation organizations, and government agencies to implement sustainable harvesting and cultivation initiatives.

   - Pool resources, share knowledge, and coordinate efforts to conserve wild goldenseal populations and promote sustainable management practices.

8. **Education and Outreach:**

   - Raise awareness about the importance of goldenseal conservation and sustainable harvesting practices among stakeholders, including harvesters, growers, consumers, and policymakers.

   - Provide training, educational materials, and outreach programs to promote responsible stewardship of goldenseal and its natural habitats.

9. **Policy Support:**

   - Advocate for policies and regulations that support sustainable harvesting, cultivation, and conservation of goldenseal and other wild medicinal plants.

   - Engage policymakers, legislators, and regulatory agencies to enact measures that protect wild populations and promote sustainable management practices.

By adopting sustainable harvesting and cultivation practices, we can help conserve wild goldenseal populations, protect biodiversity, and ensure the availability of this valuable medicinal plant for future generations. Through collaborative efforts and a commitment to responsible stewardship, we can support the sustainable use of goldenseal while safeguarding its natural habitats and ecological integrity.

Sources:

1. United Plant Savers. (2021). UpS Conservation Priorities: Goldenseal. Retrieved from https://unitedplantsavers.org/goldenseal-conservation-priorities/

2. Appalachian Beginning Forest Farmer Coalition. (n.d.). Goldenseal. Retrieved from https://www.beginningforestfarmer.org/goldenseal

3. Foster, S., & Chilton, L. (1995). Goldenseal (Hydrastis canadensis): Conservation Assessment for New England. Plant Conservation Alliance. Retrieved from https://www.fs.fed.us/wildflowers/ethnobotany/documents/conservation/goldenseal.pdf

4. World Wildlife Fund. (n.d.). Forest Stewardship Council (FSC). Retrieved from https://www.worldwildlife.org/initiatives/forest-stewardship-council-fsc

Chapter 35: Advocating for the Protection of Goldenseal's Habitat

Goldenseal (Hydrastis canadensis) is a valuable medicinal plant native to North America, but its natural habitat faces numerous threats, including habitat loss, deforestation, urban development, and climate change. Protecting the habitat of goldenseal is essential for conserving wild populations and ensuring the long-term survival of this culturally and ecologically significant plant. In this chapter, we'll explore strategies for advocating for the protection of goldenseal's habitat and promoting conservation efforts.

1. **Habitat Conservation Initiatives:**
   - Support and participate in habitat conservation initiatives aimed at protecting and restoring the natural habitats of goldenseal.
   - Advocate for the establishment of protected areas, conservation easements, and wildlife corridors to safeguard critical habitats for goldenseal and other native species.

2. **Land Use Planning and Zoning:**
   - Advocate for responsible land use planning and zoning regulations that prioritize the conservation of natural habitats and biodiversity.
   - Encourage sustainable development practices, green infrastructure, and smart growth policies to minimize the impact on goldenseal habitat.

3. **Public Awareness and Education:**

- Raise public awareness about the importance of goldenseal habitat conservation through education, outreach, and advocacy campaigns.

- Engage local communities, landowners, policymakers, and stakeholders in discussions about the value of preserving natural habitats and the benefits of biodiversity conservation.

4. **Collaboration with Stakeholders:**

- Collaborate with landowners, farmers, foresters, and other stakeholders to develop conservation agreements, stewardship programs, and voluntary conservation measures.

- Foster partnerships and alliances with diverse stakeholders to leverage resources, share expertise, and implement effective conservation strategies.

5. **Research and Monitoring:**

- Support scientific research and monitoring efforts to assess the status of goldenseal populations, identify threats to habitat integrity, and inform conservation priorities.

- Collect data on habitat characteristics, population dynamics, and ecological interactions to guide conservation planning and management decisions.

6. **Policy Advocacy:**

   - Advocate for policies and legislation that protect and conserve the habitat of goldenseal and other native plants.

   - Lobby lawmakers, government agencies, and regulatory bodies to enact measures that promote habitat conservation, sustainable land management, and biodiversity protection.

7. **Restoration and Rehabilitation:**

   - Support habitat restoration and rehabilitation projects aimed at enhancing the quality and resilience of goldenseal habitat.

   - Volunteer for tree planting, stream restoration, invasive species removal, and other habitat improvement activities to restore degraded ecosystems and promote biodiversity.

8. **Conservation Funding and Grants:**

   - Advocate for increased funding and grants for habitat conservation projects, research initiatives, and land acquisition efforts.

   - Seek financial support from government agencies, private foundations, philanthropic organizations, and conservation grants programs to fund habitat protection and restoration activities.

9. **Long-Term Planning and Adaptation:**

   - Develop long-term conservation plans and adaptation strategies to address the impacts of climate change, habitat fragmentation, and other emerging threats to goldenseal habitat.

   - Incorporate principles of resilience, connectivity, and ecosystem-based management into conservation planning to enhance the capacity of habitats to withstand environmental challenges.

By advocating for the protection of goldenseal's habitat and championing conservation efforts, we can help preserve this valuable medicinal plant for future generations and maintain the ecological integrity of its native ecosystems.

Sources:

1. United States Fish and Wildlife Service. (n.d.). Native Plants for Wildlife Habitat and Conservation Landscaping: Goldenseal (Hydrastis canadensis). Retrieved from https://www.fws.gov/wildflower/native-plants/goldenseal.html

2. United Plant Savers. (2021). Goldenseal Conservation Concerns. Retrieved from https://unitedplantsavers.org/goldenseal-conservation-concerns/

3. Appalachian Beginning Forest Farmer Coalition. (n.d.). Goldenseal. Retrieved from https://www.beginningforestfarmer.org/goldenseal

4. Missouri Botanical Garden. (n.d.). Hydrastis canadensis. Retrieved from http://www.missouribotanicalgarden.org/PlantFinder/PlantFinderDetails.aspx?kempercode=c550

Chapter 36: Embracing Goldenseal as a Key Player in Natural Health Care

Goldenseal (Hydrastis canadensis) holds immense potential as a key player in natural healthcare, offering a wide range of therapeutic benefits and applications. From its traditional use by indigenous cultures to its modern-day popularity as a medicinal herb, goldenseal has earned recognition for its effectiveness in promoting health and wellness. In this chapter, we'll explore the role of goldenseal as a cornerstone of natural healthcare and its contributions to holistic healing practices.

1. Traditional Wisdom and Indigenous Knowledge:

- Honor the rich tradition of goldenseal use by indigenous cultures, who valued the plant for its healing properties and spiritual significance.

- Draw inspiration from traditional healing practices and indigenous knowledge systems that recognize the holistic nature of health and wellness.

2. Botanical Medicine and Herbal Remedies:

- Embrace goldenseal as a cornerstone of botanical medicine and herbal remedies, harnessing its therapeutic properties to address a variety of health concerns.

- Incorporate goldenseal into herbal formulations, tinctures, teas, salves, and other preparations to support holistic healing and promote overall well-being.

3. **Preventive Healthcare and Wellness Promotion:**

- Promote the use of goldenseal as part of a preventive healthcare regimen to support immune function, enhance resilience, and maintain vitality.

- Educate individuals about the benefits of integrating goldenseal into their daily wellness routines to prevent illness, promote longevity, and optimize health outcomes.

4. **Complementary and Integrative Medicine:**

- Advocate for the integration of goldenseal into complementary and integrative medicine practices, which combine conventional and natural approaches to healthcare.

- Collaborate with healthcare providers, naturopathic physicians, herbalists, and other practitioners to incorporate goldenseal into comprehensive treatment plans for patients.

5. **Evidence-Based Medicine and Scientific Research:**

- Support scientific research efforts to explore the efficacy, safety, and mechanisms of action of goldenseal in various health conditions.

- Advocate for evidence-based medicine practices that rely on empirical data and clinical research to inform decision-making and treatment recommendations.

6. **Sustainable Sourcing and Responsible Harvesting:**

- Promote sustainable sourcing practices and responsible harvesting methods to ensure the long-term viability of wild goldenseal populations.

- Encourage the cultivation of goldenseal using organic and regenerative farming techniques to minimize environmental impact and support ethical sourcing.

7. **Public Education and Awareness:**

- Raise public awareness about the health benefits of goldenseal and its role in natural healthcare through educational campaigns, workshops, and community outreach initiatives.

- Provide accurate and accessible information about goldenseal's medicinal properties, therapeutic uses, and safety considerations to empower individuals to make informed healthcare choices.

8. **Advocacy for Herbal Medicine and Plant Conservation:**

- Advocate for the recognition and integration of herbal medicine into mainstream healthcare systems, promoting greater access to natural remedies and botanical therapies.

- Support initiatives and organizations dedicated to plant conservation, biodiversity protection, and the preservation of medicinal plant species like goldenseal.

By embracing goldenseal as a key player in natural healthcare and promoting its use in holistic healing practices, we can harness the plant's therapeutic potential to promote health, vitality, and well-being for individuals and communities worldwide.

Sources:

1. World Health Organization. (2013). Traditional Medicine Strategy 2014-2023. Retrieved from https://www.who.int/medicines/publications/traditiona l/trm_strategy14_23/en/

2. United Plant Savers. (2021). Goldenseal Conservation Concerns. Retrieved from https://unitedplantsavers.org/goldenseal-conservation-concerns/

3. American Herbalists Guild. (n.d.). About Herbal Medicine. Retrieved from https://www.americanherbalistsguild.com/about-herbal -medicine